Classifications in Facial Plastic Surgery

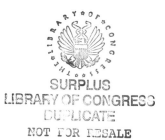

Classifications in Facial Plastic Surgery

Paul J. Oxley

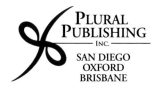

PLURAL
PUBLISHING
INC.

SAN DIEGO
OXFORD
BRISBANE

PLURAL PUBLISHING
INC.

5521 Ruffin Road
San Diego, CA 92123

e-mail: info@pluralpublishing.com
Web site: http://www.pluralpublishing.com

49 Bath Street
Abingdon, Oxfordshire OX14 1EA
United Kingdom

Typeset in 10½/13 Garamond by Flanagan's Publishing Services, Inc.
Printed in Malaysia by Four-Colour Print Group

Library of Congress Cataloging-in-Publication Data:

Oxley, Paul James.
   Classifications in facial plastic surgery / Paul James Oxley.
        p. ; cm.
   Includes bibliographical references and index.
   ISBN-13: 978-1-59756-185-3 (alk. paper)
   ISBN-10: 1-59756-185-1 (alk. paper)
   1. Face—Surgery. 2. Surgery, Plastic.
   [DNLM: 1. Face—surgery. 2. Reconstructive Surgical Procedures—classification.
3. Stomatognathic Diseases—surgery. WE 15 O98c 2008] I. Title.
   RD523.O95 2008
   617.5'20592—dc22
                                                    2008018649

Contents

Foreword

To classify is to create order in our lives. Arranging facts, features, and observations is critical to the acquisition of knowledge. The biological definition of "classification" is the systematic arrangement of living organisms in categories based upon natural relationships—the most famous is Linnaeus's *Systema Naturae*. Although medical students usually forget Linnaean taxonomy, they learn to classify in an effort to organize and memorize what seems important in the daily downpour of new information. Who has forgotten that the autonomic nervous system is divided into the parasympathetic and the sympathetic? Who does not remember how to mentally scroll the etiology of disease as either congenital, inflammatory (infectious), metabolic, neoplastic, post-traumatic, or degenerative?

During residency and practice, this habit of classifying continues in the care of patients. Dr. Paul Oxley has compiled a reference text of 100 classifications that apply to the surgical treatment of acquired and congenital disorders in the head and neck. Following each classification and pertinent citations, Dr. Oxley gives a short explanation and, in many entries, he relinquishes the page to a guest expert for further commentary. These remarks read easily and range from congratulatory, circumspect, and controversial to critical.

Few classifications withstand the scrutiny of application. Experienced clinicians recognize the limitations of these mental constructs. Wizened surgeons know that there are gray or overlapping areas in most systems and many patients do not fit comfortably in a particular slot. With advances in biomedical science and technology, even the best of systems will need modification, whereas others will wither from desuetude and be abandoned. Dear reader, you must decide which classifications are useful.

John B. Mulliken, M.D.
Boston, Massachusetts

Preface

As a resident in Plastic Surgery there were many times when I was asked to classify a given clinical situation. Research projects often demanded a classifying system to define or measure the problem in question. My qualifying exam had numerous questions relating to classification systems. The biggest challenge wasn't learning the system, it was finding the system. There was no good source that focused on classification systems in a clear and concise fashion.

Dr. Patty Clugston once asked me to classify NOE fractures while we tried to repair a facial smash. I happily recited the one found in this book. All she said was that she wanted "the other one," so after finishing the case I spent a couple of hours trying to find another classification of NOE fractures. I finally found one by Dr. Joe Gruss of Seattle, but the frustration of looking for such a long time reinforced the need for a better source.

The first major question with any classification system is why is it there? Classifying things is something that we are trained to do from a very early age. Whether it is the four food groups or a person's hair color, we quickly learn to identify people or things as members of certain groups. Obviously in some circumstances this is wrong, but that is a political discussion best had elsewhere. But why do we classify things? Simply put, classifying things makes them easier to understand, remember, or act upon.

Medicine is no different than any other field. The first thing one learns in Pathology is to identify things as to the source of the pathology. For example, at the University of British Columbia we learned the mnemonic VINDICATTE: Vascular, Infectious, Neoplastic, Degenerative, Iatrogenic/Idiopathic, Congenital, Autoimmune, Toxic/Metabolic, Traumatic, and Endocrine. From this, further classifications are learned to better define certain conditions.

Plastic Surgery has classifications in all areas, from hand surgery to cosmetic. In Facial Plastic and Reconstructive Surgery, there are many ways of looking at each area of the head and neck. For example, one can look at things anatomically, etiologically, or clinically (treatment or prognostic). Some classifications are known by the names that created them and are "universally" understood. Le Fort fractures and Tessier facial clefts are examples of these eponymous systems. Indeed, there are many more classifications than those presented in this book. I tried to choose commonly used classifications, some good and some bad, and tried to elucidate their strengths and weakness.

The next question then is what makes a good classification? A good classification needs to be easy to apply, objective in nature to allow greater reproducibility between users, and must present the information in a clearly understood manner. The best ones tend to be intuitive, simple, and relevant. The easy ones to remember tend to become more severe or more complex as one moves up the system. Dr. Brian Peterson relies on the branching flow chart as the best type of classification, starting broadly and becoming more refined.

Some classifications use numbers or letters to convey their information, others depend on words. Words are great for lesser used systems but tend to take more time or space to convey the information. Numbers or letters are ideal but are useless if the recipient of the information does not know the system.

Dr. Kevin Bush, one of my professors while I was a Resident, used to torment us by wanting more from us than just rote memorization of a system. He actually wanted us to understand the system and in what situations it would be useful. After a few blank stares, we slowly learned that classifications need to convey information of a certain type to be of use in one of the following ways: Description, Diagnosis, Etiology, Treatment, Prognosis, or Research.

Let me give a very simple example. If I told you that someone was redheaded, that is purely descriptive or diagnostic as it conveys no information about gender, age, hair length, baldness, or any other physical characteristics of the hair or the person to whom it belongs. But does it have any secondary uses, such as in research? A research friendly classification is best if it is purely objective. Therefore, the hair color system is clear enough to be applied to research, for example, if one wanted to look at skin cancer rates between people with red versus brown hair. The problem now is that this is not a very precise classification. Where do you put people with reddish brown hair?

This book presents almost 100 classifications pertaining to Facial Plastic and Reconstructive Surgery. Each is presented with its original citation where possible or a citation of a source that I found particularly useful. I encourage students who wish to understand more of the clinical information around a given classification to refer to these sources. Some references also contain treatment algorithms that are not repeated in this text as that was not the intention of this book.

As you will see, anything can be classified in more than one way, and people are forever trying to simplify or expand the work done previously by others. Sometimes this works, other times it leaves the user even more confused than before. Cleft lip and palate can be classified by etiology, whether it is in isolation or in the presence of a syndrome or sequence, anatomic location, the tissues involved, severity or complexity, and treatment options utilized. So which system does one use?

Often, it is best to just describe what you see if uncertain. However, when a clear, concise method of conveying that information exists, this is when clinicians start using classifying systems.

If you have classification systems that you find useful and were not included in this book, please forward them to me. Also, if you strongly disagree with any of the evaluations or comments on these systems, please let me know as well. Perhaps these could be included in future editions of this text.

Paul J. Oxley, MD, FRCSC
Vancouver, Canada, June, 2008

Acknowledgments

I would like to thank all my professors who inspired me to write this book, as well as my parents and all of the residents, past and present, who encouraged me to write it.

I also want to thank the guest authors whose comments were invaluable additions to this book. Their knowledge is greatly appreciated, as was the time they spent helping make this book what it is.

Finally, I want to thank my wife Calla, without whose help and patience this book would never have become a reality.

Paul J. Oxley

Contributors

Oleh M. Antonyshyn, MD, FRCSC
Assistant Professor, Division of Plastic
    Surgery
Sunnybrook and Women's College
    Health Sciences Centre
University of Toronto
Toronto, Ontario
Chapter 8

Kevin L. Bush, MD, FRCSC
Clinical Associate Professor
Division of Plastic Surgery
University of British Columbia
Vancouver, British Columbia
Chapters 3 and 8

Nicholas J. Carr, MD, FRCSC
Clinical Associate Professor
Head, Division of Plastic Surgery
University of British Columbia
Vancouver, British Columbia
Chapters 1, 4, and 8

**Douglas J. Courtemanche, MD, MS,
FRCSC**
Clinical Associate Professor
British Columbia's Children's Hospital
University of British Columbia
Vancouver, British Columbia
Chapters, 1, 3, 8, and 9

**Richard Crawford, MD, FRCPC
(Gen Path, Anat Path, Dermatology)**
Clinical Professor
Departments of Dermatology and
    Pathology
University of British Columbia
Vancouver, British Columbia
Chapters 2 and 4

Donald M. P. Guichon, MD, FRCSC
Plastic Surgeon
Surrey, British Columbia
Chapters 4 and 5

**Navraj Singh Heran, BSc, MD,
FRCSC**
Neurosurgeon
Fraser Health Authority
British Columbia
Chapters 3 and 8

Martin Jugenburg, MD, FRCSC
Microsurgery Fellow
Sloan Kettering Memorial Cancer
    Center
New York, New York
Chapters 2 and 7

Don Lalonde, MD, FRCSC
Professor
Division of Plastic Surgery
Dalhousie University
St. John, New Brunswick
Chapter 3

Adrian T. Lee, MD, FRCSC
Plastic Surgeon
Surrey, British Columbia
Chapter 7

Perry Liu, MD
Fellow
Medical College Chang Gung University
    Chang Gung Memorial Hospital
Taipei, Taiwan, ROC
Chapter 7

Colleeen McCarthy, MD, MSc, FRCSC
Assistant Attending Surgeon
Plastic and Reconstructive Surgery
Sloan Kettering Memorial Cancer
  Center
New York, New York
Chapters 2 and 7

Rizwan A. Mian, MD, MS, FRCSC
Clinical Instructor
Division of Plastic Surgery
University of British Columbia
Vancouver, British Columbia
Chapter 8

John B. Mulliken, MD
Professor of Surgery
Harvard Medical School
Boston, Massachusetts
Foreword

David Naysmith, BSc, DMD, MD, FRCSC
Clinical Instructor
Division of Plastic Surgery
University of British Columbia
Victoria, British Columbia
Chapter 5

Paul J. Oxley, BSc, MD, FRCSC
Clinical Instructor
Division of Plastic Surgery
University of British Columbia
Vancouver, British Columbia
Chapters 1-9

Andrea L. Pusic, MD, MHS, FRCSC
Assistant Attending Surgeon
Plastic and Reconstructive Surgery
Sloan Kettering Memorial Cancer
  Center
New York, New York
Chapters 2 and 7

Oscar M. Ramirez, MD, FACS
Clinical Assistant Professor
Johns Hopkins University School of
  Medicine
University of Maryland School of
  Medicine
Baltimore, Maryland
Chapters 3 and 4

Paul L. Schnur, MD
Assistant Professor and Chair
Division of Plastic Surgery
Mayo Medical School
Scottsdale, Arizona
Chapter 4

Charles F. T. Snelling, MD, FRCSC
Former Director BC Professional
  Firefighters Burn Unit
Professor Emeritus
University of British Columbia
Vancouver, British Columbia
Chapters 7 and 8

Edward E. Tredget, MD, MSc, FRCSC
Professor of Plastic Surgery
University of Alberta
Edmonton, Alberta
Chapter 8

Luis O. Vasconez, MD
Professor of Plastic Surgery
University of Alabama, Birmingham
Birmingham, Alabama
Chapter 4, 5, and 9

Cindy Verchere, MD, FRCSC
Clinical Assistant Professor
British Columbia's Childrens'
  Hospital
University of British Columbia
Vancouver, British Columbia
Chapters 1 and 3

Robyn Watts, BSc, MD, FRCSC
Plastic Surgeon
Richmond, British Columbia
Chapter 8

Fu-Chan Wei, MD, FACS
Professor of Plastic Surgery
Dean, Medical College Chang Gung
    University

Chang Gung Memorial Hospital
Taipei, Taiwan, ROC
Chapter 7

Gordon Wilkes, MD, FRCSC
Clinical Professor of Plastic Surgery
University of Alberta
Edmonton, Alberta
Chapter 3

To Pierce

Chapter 1

ACQUIRED

Ectropion

What It Classifies

Ectropion based on the degree of cosmetic and functional consequences.

System

See Table 1–1.

Table 1–1. Ectropion

Grade	Description
1	Punctal ectropion: lower punctum pointing upward away from globe.
2	Visible, partially everted eyelid with scleral show
3	Conjunctival hyperemia with gross mucosal thickening
4	Same as 4 but with exposure keratitis

Ectropion associated with epiphora denoted with letter "s"—eg, 2s

Source: From "Ectropion following excision of lower eyelid tumours and full thickness skin graft repair," by Rubin P, Mykula R, Griffiths RW. *Br J Plast Surg.* 2005;58 pp. 353–360. Copyright 2005 by Lippincott, Williams & Wilkins. Reprinted with permission.

Reference

Rubin P, Mykula R, Griffiths RW. Ectropion following excision of lower eyelid tumours and full thickness skin graft repair. *Br J Plast Surg.* 2005;58:353–360.

Uses

Primary: Description, Diagnosis

Secondary: Treatment, Research

Limited/none: Prognosis, Etiology

Comments

Dr. Paul Oxley

Acquired ectropion is usually a complication of an operation on the lower eyelid as well as a natural occurrence with age. This classification describes the condition from the point of view of the degree of changes seen not only to the eyelid but also to the eye itself. The "s" modifier is a useful addition so as to identify those patients with epiphora as this bothersome condition can occur with any degree of ectropion.

It does not specifically comment on the cause of the condition that can have a significant impact on the corrective procedure of choice. Indeed, in many cases in the immediate postoperative period, minor ectropion is best dealt with by local care such as natural tears, massage, and reassurance.

Möbius Syndrome

What It Classifies

Categorization and scoring of Möbius syndrome.

AKA

CLUFT System

System

See Table 1–2.

Reference

Abramson DL, Cohen MM Jr, Mulliken JB. Möbius syndrome: classification and grading system. *Plast Reconstr Surg.* 1998; 102(4):961–967.

Uses

Primary: Description, Research, Diagnosis

Secondary: Treatment

Limited/none: Prognosis, Etiology

Comments

Dr. Paul Oxley

Möbius syndrome is an uncommon disorder of unknown etiology that affects the face and facial nerves VI and VII, limbs, and thorax. In order to study etiology and management, cooperation between multiple institutions is required to obtain sufficient numbers. By grading such a disorder it allows clear description of the condition, easy comparison between sites and management techniques, and gathering of a large enough study population to begin studies of pathogenesis.

This system was designed to help categorize and compare the different patients for phenotype and outcome purposes. After studying 27 patients the authors devised a scoring system for not only the cranial nerve deficits seen in Möbius syndrome, but also the widely variable abnormalitites of the face, trunk, and limbs. The term CLUFT comes from the first letter of each affected area, with each given a score of 0 to 3. The number can be given after each letter. The total score is not of clinical significance when compared to the score for each component and is therefore not generally tallied up.

Table 1–2. Mobius

Anatomic Site	Score
C: Cranial nerves	
VII nerve partial	0
VI and VII partial	1
VI and VII complete	2
Additional nerve involvement	3
If bilateral and equal add	B
L: Lower extremity	
Normal	0
Talipes equinovarus, syndactyly, ankylosis	1
Absent phalanges	2
Longitudinal or transverse defects	3
U: Upper extremity	
Normal	0
Digital hypoplasia or failure of differentiation	1
Ectrodactyly	2
Failure of formation, longitudinal or transverse	3
F: Facial structural anomaly	
Normal	0
Cleft palate	1
Micrognathia	2
Microtia, microphthalmia, abnormal joint, etc	3
T: Thorax	
Normal	0
Scoliosis	1
Pectoral hypoplasia or breast anomaly	2
Chest wall deformity, breast or pectoral Aplasia	3

Source: From "Möbius syndrome: classification and grading system," Abramson DL, Cohen MM Jr, Mulliken JB. *Plast Reconstr Surg.* 1998;102(4): 961–967. Copyright 1998 by Lippincott, Williams & Wilkins. Reprinted with permission.

Dr. Cindy Verchere

I found this classification to be too bulky to use with clinical ease, although in a study situation, or in a clinical database (for which I believe it was designed), it would provide very complete information about an individual patient, and may allow better comparisons between patients. I'm not sure that the number in each subgroup is meant to represent severity; is scoliosis less severe than pectoral hypoplasia, for example, or micrognathia less severe than cleft palate? Comparison of "scores" may be invalid—it may be more helpful as a descriptive database.

It is also a comprehensive list of possible findings that may guide a physical examination more thoroughly for those less familiar with the syndrome.

Nasal Septum Deviation

What It Classifies

The extent and pattern of deviation of the nasal septum.

System

See Table 1-3.

Reference

Guyuron B, Uzzo CD, Scull H. A practical classification of septonasal deviation and an effective guide to septal surgery. *Plast Reconstr Surg.* 1999;104(7):2202-2209.

Uses

Primary: Description, Diagnosis, Treatment

Secondary: Research

Limited/none: Etiology, Prognosis

Comments

Dr. Paul Oxley

Septal deviation can lead to breathing difficulties, sinus or ear infections, or cosmetic changes (Fig 1-1). Many different techniques exist to correct the septum.

Table 1-3. Nasal Septal Deviation

Type	Description
Type I:	Septal tilt • No curve • Tilted to one side of the nose anteriorly and to the opposite side posteriorly, • Maxillary crest remained straight
Type II:	C-shaped, anteroposterior deviation • Maxillary crest and nasal spine also deviated
Type III:	C-shaped cephalocaudal • Similar to Type II except for direction of curve
Type IV:	S-shaped anteroposterior • Two curvatures next to each other in opposing directions
Type V:	S-shaped cephalocaudal • Similar to Type IV
Type VI:	Localized deviations or large spurs

Source: From "A practical classification of septonasal deviation and an effective guide to septal surgery" Guyuron B, Uzzo CD, Scull H. *Plast Reconstr Surg.* 1999;104(7), pp. 2202–2209. Copyright 1999 by Lippincott, Williams & Wilkins. Reprinted with permission.

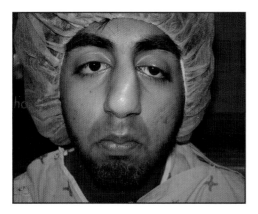

Fig 1–1. Severe posttraumatic nasal deviation.

for reconstruction. They believe that applying one surgical technique to each type of deviation may lead to unsatisfactory results. For that reason they devised this problem-oriented classification and suggest treatments for each. These treatment recommendations are found in the original article.

When one understands the anatomy and subsequent pathology any procedure is better performed. For this reason, this is a very useful system that can be applied to help diagnose, describe and suggest treatment options.

Dr. Nick Carr

The concern for any surgeon is in selecting the best procedure for the deviation encountered.

The authors reviewed 93 septal surgeries and describe 6 types of septal deviation requiring different techniques

This is an intuitively obvious classification that does lead to some sound treatment recommendations and establishes the important principle that not all deviated septums should be treated in the same fashion.

TMJ Disk Disease

What It Classifies

Physical symptoms related to varying degrees of temporomandibular joint (TMJ) degeneration.

System

I (Early)

No change in ROM, occasional grinding or clicking, no deformity, slight anterior displacement of disk.

II (Early/intermediate)

No change in ROM, sticks and clicks, occasional pain, slight deformity, normal bone, anterior displacement of disk.

III (Intermediate)

Decreased ROM, sticks and clicks, painful, anteriorly displaced, thickening of disk, normal bone.

IV (Intermediate/late)

Hypermobility and subluxation, painful, abnormal bone, thick disk, adhesions may be present.

V (late)

Dislocatable, painful, limited ROM, perforated disk, adhesions present. Joint crepitus and degenerative bone changes.

Reference

Wilkes CH. Internal derangements of the temperomandibular joint. Pathological varia-tions. *Arch Otolaryngol Head Neck Surg.* 1989;115:469. Copyright 1989 by the American Medical Association. All rights reserved. Reprinted with permission.

Uses

Primary: Description, Diagnosis

Secondary: Treatment, Prognosis, Etiology

Limited/none: Research

Comments

Dr. Paul Oxley

The TMJ disk is located between the head of the condyle and the mandibular fossa, making it susceptible to significant pressure and repetitive forces. Grinding of the teeth, although a common cause of TMJ pathology, is not seen in all patients with significant joint disease. Over time, some people experience degenerative arthritis of this joint, causing pain and clicking or locking.

The symptoms related to TMJ disease do not readily correlate with the physical findings or radiologic changes. This is a common finding in degenerative diseases of most joints. Some will have essentially no symptoms until very late stage disease, whereas others present earlier in the disease process. This classification represents the common presentation of TMJ degenerative disk disease.

This is a slightly cumbersome classification that covers overall pathology of the TMJ. It is able to provide some help in directing treatment options, though these options are limited in many cases. Prognosis is variable by age and etiology of the problem.

Dr. Doug Courtemanche

The importance of this staging system is that it is based on a very large number of observations with correlation between clinical observations, imaging, operative findings, and pathology. The system details the stages of progression in patients with internal derangement of the TMJ from benign, intermittent clicking with no other symptoms to debilitating end stage osteoarthritis. Even with 540 procedures on 740 joints the author is unable to comment on the time course of the disease or the risk of progressing from one stage to the next over time. This is due to the high degree of variability in the disease process. It is important to recognize that this is a disease that affects young women.

The paper focuses on disk pathomechanics and does not comment on other factors in the etiology of TMJ disease such as steep articular eminence anatomy, which might predispose to early disk degeneration.

Chapter 2

CANCER

What It Classifies

The anatomic location of lymph nodes in the head and neck using a numerical designation.

System

See Table 2-1.

Table 2-1. Cervical Lymph Nodes

Level	Location
I	Submandibular and submental nodes (all nodes in floor of mouth)
II	Internal jugular chain (or deep cervical chain) nodes —nodes about internal jugular vein from skull base to hyoid bone (same level as carotid bifurcation)
III	Nodes about internal jugular vein from hyoid bone to cricoid cartilage (same level that omohyoid muscle crosses internal jugular chain)
IV	Infraomohyoid nodes about internal jugular vein between cricoid cartilage and supraclavicular fossa
V	Posterior triangle nodes (deep to sternocleidomastoid muscle)
VI	Nodes related to thyroid gland
VII	Nodes in tracheoesophageal groove, about esophagus extending down to superior mediastinum

Source: From Som PM. "Lymph nodes of the neck." *Radiology*, 1987;165:593. Copyright 1987 by the Radiological Society of North America. Reprinted with permission.

Reference

Som PM. Lymph nodes of the neck. *Radiology.* 1987;165:593.

Uses

Primary: Research, Description

Secondary: Diagnosis

Limited/none: Etiology, Prognosis, Treatment

Comments

Dr. Paul J. Oxley

The presence of nodal involvement in cancer of the head and neck has always had a significant influence on the subsequent treatment and prognosis. The location of the lymph nodes has historically been done by using anatomic terms, such as originally described by Rouviere. In order to simplify the recording of these locations, a numeric system has been widely used over the past 20 years. This takes the anatomic locations and assigns a number to them. This can be used clinically and radiologically to describe the location of the affected nodes.

The exact diagnosis of nodal involvement can only be made after histologic sampling of the tissue, as enlarged lymph nodes may be reactive to inflammation or infection about the tumor. The treatment then depends on how many nodes are present, whether they are ipsilateral or bilateral, the tissue type of the tumor, and patient factors such as age and comorbid conditions.

This system is a good one for students to learn as it simplifies the different areas of the cervical nodes. Each area of the head and neck tends to drain to specific areas of the cervical lymph nodes. This knowledge can be useful for helping to find the location of an unknown primary in the face of node positive disease.

Breslow's Classification of Melanoma Depth

What It Classifies

Absolute depth of invasion of a Malignant Melanoma.

System

Original

Level I	<0.75 mm deep
Level II	0.76 to 1.5 mm deep
Level III	1.6 to 3.0 mm deep
Level IV	>3.0 mm deep

Modified

Level I	<1.00 mm deep
Level II	1.01 to 2.00 mm deep
Level III	2.01 to 4.00 mm deep
Level IV	>4.01 mm deep

(Please see Fig 2-3 in the next section.)

References

Balch CM, et al. Final version of the American Joint Committee on Cancer staging system for cutaneous melanoma. *J Clin Oncol.* 2001;19(16):3635-3648.

Breslow A. Thickness, cross-sectional areas and depth of invasion in the prognosis of cutaneous melanoma. *Ann Surg.* 1970; 171(5):902-908.

Seigler HF. Surgical management of cutaneous melanoma. In: Georgiade GS, Riefkohl R & Levin LS, eds. *Georgiade Plastic, Max-illofacial and Reconstructive Surgery,* 3rd ed. Baltimore, Md: Williams & Wilkins; 1997:193.

Solky BA, Mihm MC, Tsao H, Sober A. Factors influencing survival in melanoma patients. In: Rigel DS, Friedman RJ, Dzubow LM, et al, eds. *Cancer of the Skin.* Philadelphia, Pa: Elsevier Saunders; 2005:189-202.

Uses

Primary: Prognosis, Diagnosis, Treatment, Research

Secondary: Description

Limited/none: Etiology

Comments

Dr. Paul Oxley

The Breslow classification was the first widely accepted system that recognized absolute depth of invasion as an important determinant of survival in patients with melanoma. Other systems, such as Clark's depth, is based on histopathologic depth. The two systems work well together. Depending on the location of the melanoma on the body, one system may be more influential in the prognosis than the other. For example, a 2-mm deep melanoma on an eyelid is more likely to invade into deep tissue than a similar depth melanoma on the back.

The original Breslow classification system has been replaced by a similar but more widely accepted scale that uses slightly different cutoffs. Most centers now use modified levels of less than 1 mm, 1 to 2 mm, 2 to 4 mm, and greater than 4 mm as the level of invasion, with treatment, staging, and prognosis depending on those numbers (Figs 2–1 and 2–2).

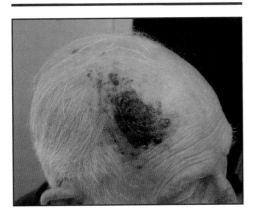

Fig 2–1. 8-mm deep, Clark's level V melanoma.

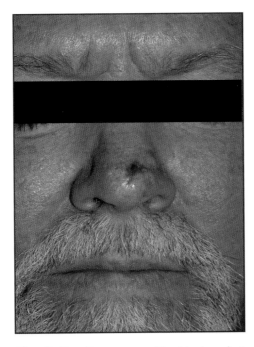

Fig 2–2. Recurrent Clark's level 1 melanoma

Dr. Richard Crawford

The full range of Breslow depth is the most significant prognostic factor within the melanoma primary tumor. It has the greatest influence of any factor on subsequent decisions about width of local excision, the option of sentinel node biopsy, and the potential indication to investigate for distant metastases. Older studies investigating prognostic significance were based on the "Original" classification, but recent studies as well as TNM classification, staging, and management decisions are all based on the "Modified" version.

Mode of biopsy may complicate interpretation of the Breslow depth. It is most reliably and efficiently assessed by complete excision rather than partial biopsy of a melanoma. If a melanoma is initially assessed by a partial incisional biopsy, such as a punch biopsy, then the Breslow depth that is measured within the tissue submitted to the pathologist is likely to underestimate the Breslow thickness measured when the entire lesion is excised, because a partial biopsy is likely, by chance, to miss sampling the deepest extent of the melanoma. Even worse, if a melanoma is sampled by a shave biopsy and the incision cuts horizontally through the tumor, then the ability to accurately measure the depth is lost forever; it is not geometrically valid to arithmetically sum the thickness on a sequence of two biopsies in an effort to correct this error.

Unusual aspects of the tumor may also complicate the pathologist's effort to report a depth. These include ulceration, partial regression, or extension of tumor horizontally from the deep portion of skin adnexal structures. Approaches to these difficult situations have been standardized. Because Breslow depth is such an important prognostic factor, it is often in the patient's interest to have such difficult tumors reviewed by an oncologic pathologist or a dermatopathologist.

Most pathologists report Breslow depth as an absolute measurement (for example, 1.20 mm), rather than as a level (for example level II). The levels in the Breslow classification do not correspond at all to Clark's levels, and reporting the Breslow depth as a level could lead to confusion.

Clark's Classification of Melanoma Depth

What It Classifies

The histologic depth of invasion of a Malignant Melanoma.

System

Level I	Confined to epidermis

Level II	Invades the papillary dermis but does not fill and expand it.
Level III	Expands and fills the papillary dermis
Level IV	Invades into reticular dermis
Level V	Invades into subcutaneous tissue

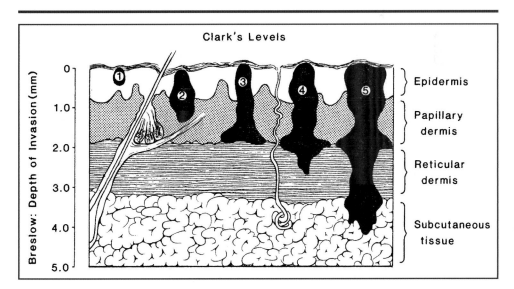

Fig 2–3. Clark and Breslow levels. From: Seigler HF, Surgical management of cutaneous melanoma. In: Georgiade GS, Riefkohl R & Levin LS, eds. *Georgiade Plastic, Maxillofacial and Reconstructive Surgery.* 3rd ed. Baltimore, Md: Williams & Wilkins; 1997, p. 195. Copyright 1997 by Lippincott, Williams & Wilkins. Reprinted with permission.

References

Balch CM, Murad TM, Soong SJ, Ingalls AL, Halpern NB, Maddox WA. A multifactorial analysis of melanoma: prognostic histopathological features comparing Clark's and Breslow's staging methods. *Ann Surg.* 1978;188(6):732–742.

Clark, WH Jr. from Bernadino EA, et al. The histogenesis and biologic behaviour of primary human malignant melanomas of the skin. *Cancer Res.* 1969; 29:705.

Massi G, LeBoit PE. *Histological Diagnosis of Nevi and Melanoma.* Wurzburg: Steinkopff Verlag Darmstadt; 2004:647.

Seigler HF. Surgical management of cutaneous melanoma. In: Georgiade GS, Riefkohl R & Levin, LS, eds. *Georgiade Plastic, Maxillofacial and Reconstructive Surgery.* 3rd ed. Baltimore, Md: Williams and Wilkins; 1997:193.

Uses

Primary: Description, Diagnosis

Secondary: Research, Treatment, Prognosis

Limited/none: Etiology

Comments

Dr. Paul Oxley

The treatment and prognosis of melanoma is based largely on the depth of invasion. This classification system standardized the depth of invasion based on the histologic extension of the tumor. Although the other major scheme, the Breslow classification, has been modified over time, the Clark classification system is still widely quoted using its original format by most pathologists in describing the tumor.

The three main factors for determining prognosis and treatment are depth of invasion in millimeters, the presence of cutaneous ulceration as a result of the tumor, and distant metastases. The Clark's level modifies the prognosis as the higher the Clark's level, the more likely the spread of the tumor. Absolute depth of invasion is difficult to compare when looking at skin with significantly different thickness (eg, back versus eyelid).

Research, diagnosis, and prognosis of the different types of melanoma is based on other features as well, including appearance, staining, presence of satellite lesions, and invasion into structures such as lymphatic, nerves, and vessels.

Dr. Richard Crawford

Clark's level has been demonstrated to be less prognostically significant overall than the measured Breslow thickness, and therefore most staging and treatment decisions are based on Breslow measurement; however, there are a few situations in which a change in Clark's level will alter staging and management.

Clark's level I is the same as in situ melanoma, whereas Clark's level II represents invasive melanoma. In one sense this is a critical distinction, as in situ melanoma at least theoretically has no metastatic potential, whereas patients with Clark's level II or greater will need to be counseled on their risk of metastasis and mortality. In another sense, however, this distinction is redundant: the invasive or in situ status of the melanoma is already conveyed in the pathologist's diagnosis itself, as well as in the reporting of a Breslow measurement in any invasive melanoma and the lack of reporting of the Breslow measurement in in situ melanomas.

The one other situation in which Clark's level has been identified to have particular prognostic value is in thin melanomas. Specifically, Clark's level IV and V tumors behave in a distinctly worse manner than those of Clark's level III or less. Because of this, the current AJCC Staging takes into account the presence of a Clark's level IV or greater, but only in these thin melanomas. As a result of the upstaging that occurs in this specific situation, Clark's level IV status occasion-ally will provide the sole indication for sentinel node biopsy in thin melanomas.

Assessment of Clark's level shows less reproducibility than the Breslow measurement. Unfortunately, this is particularly a problem at the level of differentiating level IV from level III, where it can be critical for staging and management purposes. Therefore, it may be wise to have a second pathologist review any case in which a Clark's level IV provides the sole indication for sentinel node biopsy.

Melanoma Staging

What It Classifies

The clinical stage of malignant melanoma.

System

See Table 2-2.

References

Balch CM, Buzaid AC, Soong SJ, et al. Final version of the American Joint Committee on Cancer staging system for cutaneous melanoma. *J Clin Oncol.* 2001;19(16): 3635-3648.
Solky BA, Mihm MC, Tsao H, Sober AJ. Factors influencing survival in melanoma patients. In: Rigel DS, Friedman RJ, Dzubow LM, et al, eds. *Cancer of the Skin.* Philadelphia, Pa: Elsevier Saunders; 2005:189-202.

Uses

Primary: Diagnosis, Prognosis, Research, Description

Table 2-2. Melanoma Staging

Stage	TNM
0	Tis, N0, M0
IA	T1a, N0, M0
IB	T1b, N0, M0 T2a, N0, M0
IIA	T2b, N0, M0 T3a, N0, M0
IIB	T3b, N0, M0 T4a, N0, M0
IIC	T4b, N0, M0
IIIA	T1a-T4a, N1a or N2a, M0
IIIB	T1b-T4b, N1a or N2a, M0 T1a-T4a, N1b or N2b Any T, N2c, M0
IIIC	T1b-T4b, N1b or N2b, M0 Any T, N3, M0
IV	Any T, any N, any M

Source: From Balch CM, Buzaid AC, Soong SJ, et al, Final version of the American Joint Committee on Cancer staging system for cutaneous melanoma. *J Clin Oncol.* 2001;19(16):3635-3648.

Secondary: Treatment

Limited/none: Etiology

Comments

Dr. Paul Oxley

The staging of a tumor is crucial in determining prognosis and treatment options. For example, ulceration of the primary lesion worsens prognosis. Controversy remains over the treatment of node positive disease as well as how aggressively one should look for involvement for T1-3 tumors. Treatment at many agencies also depends on patient age and comorbid conditions.

Dr. Richard Crawford

Examination of this staging system reveals a simple underlying concept:

Stage 0 = in situ disease only, without significant risk of mortality

Stages I & II = primary tumor only (45-95% 5-year survival depending on substage)

Stage III = nodal, in-transit or satellite metastases (25-70% 5-year survival)

Stage IV = distant metastases (less than 20% 5-year survival).

The large-scale prognostic studies that were used to develop this current AJCC staging system identified that the presence of ulceration conveyed an adverse prognosis equivalent to a one-level increase in Breslow depth (for example, an increase from 1.00 mm to 2.00 mm, or from 2.00 mm to 4.00 mm). Close examination of the staging system reveals that the subdivisions of stage I and stage II melanomas are based on this observation. With the presence or absence of ulceration now included in staging, this results in the following approximate 5-year survivals: stage IA 95%, stage IB 90%, stage IIA 80%, stage IIB 65%, stage IIC 45%. In addition, the presence of ulceration of the primary site also upstages the subdivisions of stage III, from IIIA to IIIB or from IIIB to IIIC. Although the importance of ulceration is highlighted in current staging, the assessment of ulceration by the pathologist can be difficult. The following need to be excluded: partial-thickness epidermal erosion; ulceration due to recent biopsy; or tissue disruption that occurs during surgery or laboratory processing. Conversely, ulceration can be missed by the pathologist. If ulceration is suspected by the surgeon performing the excision, it should be noted on the surgical pathology requisition, as it will be less apparent on gross examination in the laboratory than it was while the lesion was present on the patient; appropriate sections for histology must be submitted from the affected portion of the melanoma, otherwise the presence of ulceration will not be identified pathologically, resulting in under staging and, potentially, undertreatment.

In general, definitive surgical margins surrounding the primary tumor are based solely on Breslow depth. In contrast, consideration of the option of sentinel node biopsy and other forms of metastatic workup are based on stage IB or greater, taking into account the risk factors of not only greater Breslow depth, but also ulceration or a greater Clark's level. In this respect, stage IA melanomas alone represent low-risk melanomas, and the management of stage IB melanomas resembles that of the higher risk stage II lesions.

There are prognostic factors for melanoma that have a considerable independent bearing on the likelihood of metastasis and mortality, but do not form part of the current staging system. These factors are sometimes considered in management decisions. They include lymphatic invasion, mitotic rate and, to a lesser extent, some antigenic and genetic markers. In addition, perineural invasion conveys an increased risk of local recurrence and therefore is sometimes an indication for additional measures in local control such as wider surgical margins or adjuvant radiotherapy.

TNM Classification of Malignant Melanoma

What It Classifies

Tumor characteristics with respect to depth of invasion and metastases.

System

See Table 2-3.

References

Balch CM, et al. Final version of the American Joint Committee on Cancer staging system for cutaneous melanoma. *J Clin Oncol.* 2001;19(16):3635-3648.

Solky BA, Mihm MC, Tsao H, Sober AJ. Factors influencing survival in melanoma patients. In: Rigel DS, Friedman RJ, Dzubow LM, et al, eds. *Cancer of the Skin.* Philadelphia, Pa: Elsevier Saunders; 2005:189-202.

Uses

Primary: Research, Diagnosis, Treatment, Prognosis

Secondary: Description

Limited/none: Etiology

Comments

Dr. Paul Oxley

TNM is a standard system used to describe most cancers. The system is designed to help give a standard diagnosis for a given clinical presentation, as well as help direct treatment options based on relative prognosis. It is used to determine the stage of the cancer, and it is on this stage that most prognostic tables are based.

Dr. Richard Crawford

The large majority of melanomas do not have detectable metastases at the time of diagnosis (N0M0); therefore, primary tumor (T) classification is the only relevant factor in determining prognosis and treatment in most melanomas. In the above T classification, cases of in situ melanoma ("Tis," melanoma confined to the epidermis, equivalent to Clark's level I) are most appropriately included alongside T0. In situ melanoma, when accurately diagnosed, does not have metastatic potential and does not require any metastatic workup; it is in this sense of its natural history rather than in a strict pathologic

Table 2–3. TNM Classification of Malignant Melanoma

Primary Tumor (T):

Tx	No evidence of primary tumor	
T0	Atypical melanocytic hyperplasia (not malignant)	
T1	<1.0 mm deep	
	T1a: no ulceration or Clark's level II/III	
	T1b: with ulceration or Clark's level IV/V	
T2	1.01 to 2.0 mm deep	
	T2a: no ulceration	
	T2b: with ulceration	
T3	2.01 to 4.0 mm deep	
	T3a: no ulceration	
	T3b: with ulceration	
T4	>4.0 mm deep	
	T4a: no ulceration	
	T4b: with ulceration	

Nodal Involvement (N):

Nx   Minimal requirements to assess nodes cannot be met

N0   No regional node involvement

N1   Involvement of only one regional node station; negative regional lymph nodes and <5 in-transit metastases beyond 2 cm from primary lesion
   N1a: microscopic node
   N1b: macroscopic node

N2   Any of the following: Involvement of >1 nodal station, regional nodes >5 cm in diameter or fixed, 5 or more in-transit metastases beyond 2 cm from primary lesion with regional node involvement
   N2a: microscopic nodes
   N2b: macroscopic nodes
   N2c: in-transit metastases without metastatic lymph nodes

N3   4 or more metastatic nodes, matted nodes/gross extracapsular extension, or in transit metastases with metastatic nodes

Distant Metastases (M):

Mx   Minimal requirements to assess distant metastases cannot be met

M0   No distant metastases detected

M1   Involvement of skin or subcutaneous tissue beyond the site of primary lymph node drainage
   M1a: distant skin, subcutaneous, or nodal metastases with normal LDH
   M1b: lung metastases with normal LDH

M2   Visceral metastases
   sometimes referred to as M1(c)

sense that in situ melanoma is "not malignant." The T classification of invasive melanomas (T1 to T4) is based on the combination of Breslow depth and ulceration, and the critical Breslow depths are those within the modified Breslow classification rather than the original Breslow classification. Clark's level is pertinent only in the lowest risk invasive melanomas, that is, those that lack ulceration and are in the thinnest Breslow category. Tx occurs relatively commonly in melanoma because of the phenomenon of spontaneous regression of the primary tumor; these tumors present with local, nodal, or distant metastases and thus by definition are stage III or IV, with the expected relatively poor prognosis.

Satellite metastases lie in the skin or soft tissues within 2 cm of the primary tumor, whereas in-transit metastases lie further than 2 cm from the primary tumor, between it and the draining lymph nodes. The large-scale studies of prognostic factors that led to the 2001 "Final" AJCC classification actually suggested that both satellite metastases and in-transit metastases convey an adverse prognosis similar to metaststases within lymph nodes; therefore, revised versions of the AJCC TNM classification since 2002 include satellite metastases as well as in-transit metastases in the category of N2c or N3. This resulted in the apparent paradox that features within a wide local excision can be definitive in N classification even in the absence of disease within lymph nodes (N2c due to satellite metastases). It also emphasizes the importance of careful examination of the margin tissue within the wide local excision by the pathologist, including multiple closely spaced sections at gross examination and submission of any suspicious areas for histologic examination.

Head and Neck Tumor Staging

What It Classifies

Clinical stage of oropharyngeal tumors.

System

Stage 0	Tis, N0, M0
Stage I	T1, N0, M0
Stage II	T2, N0, M0
Stage III	T3, N0, M0
	Tn, N1, M0
Stage IV	T4, N0 or N1, M0
	Any T, N2 or 3, M0
	Any T, Any N, M1

References

O'Brien JC. Head and neck I: Tumors. *Selected Readings in Plastic Surgery.* 1985;8(9).

Richards AM. The head and neck. In: Richards AM, ed. *Key Notes in Plastic Surgery.* Oxford: Blackwell Science Limited; 2002: 106–107.

Uses

Primary: Diagnosis, Research, Treatment, Prognosis

Secondary: Description

Limited/none: Etiology

Comments

Dr. Paul J. Oxley

In any cancer, staging is crucial in determining prognosis and therefore the treatment options for any given lesion. Stages are designed so higher levels have a poorer prognosis. This is true of all cancer staging systems. In addition, they all take into account the TNM system for the tumor when determining the stage. Different cancers have different criteria to be called a T1 versus a T2, but the staging comes after those distinctions are made.

Although often the main factor when determining treatment, many agencies also depend on patient age and comorbid conditions. Staging is also useful to compare results between different treatment modalities and centers.

Histologic Classification of Salivary Gland Tumors

What It Classifies

Tumor types seen in salivary glands based on the histologic component causing the tumor.

System

Type 1: Adenomas

Type 2: Carcinomas

Type 3: Nonepithelial tumors

Type 4: Malignant tumors

Type 5: Secondary tumors

Type 6: Unclassified tumors

Type 7: Tumorlike lesions

From: *Cancer,* 70(2):1992;p. 379. Copyright 1992 American Cancer Society. This material is reproduced with permission of Wiley Liss, Inc, a subsidiary of John Wiley & Sons, Inc.

References

O'Brien JC. Head and neck I: tumors. *Selected Readings in Plastic Surgery*. 1985;8(9).

Note. Portions of this section were taken from "The WHO's histological classification of salivary gland tumors. A commentary on the second edition," by Seifert G, Sobin LH, 1992 *Cancer* 70(2):379. Copyright 1992 by American Cancer Society. This material is reproduced with permission of Wiley-Liss, Inc, a subsidiary of John Wiley & Sons, Inc.

Uses

Primary: Description, Diagnosis

Secondary: Research, Etiology

Limited/none: Prognosis, Treatment

Comments

Dr. Paul Oxley

The histologic classification of salivary gland tumors is important because there is a sgnificant difference in prognosis and treatment among lesions. The majority of salivary gland tumors are benign. This classification is useful both clinically and in research. It always requires a tissue diagnosis and therefore depends on an invasive procedure. It is a useful classification for students to help them develop the framework for looking at the greater than 30 masses that are considered salivary gland tumors.

As noted above, prognosis and treatment vary by type of tumor, as well as size, local involvement, and any metastases. It will also be determined by patient factors such as co morbid conditions and age.

Dr. Richard Crawford

The pathology of salivary gland tumors is unusually complex for such a small organ. This classification does a good job of organizing a very large number of tumors into a reasonably logical sequence. The category of "malignant tumors" requires clarification. Carcinomas ("type 2") are by definition malignant tumors ("type 4"), so "type 4" refers only to noncarcinomatous malignant tumors, such as sarcomas and lymphomas. Nonepithelial tumors ("type 3") that also happen to be malignant ("type 4") are most appropriate classified for prognostic and treatment purposes along with other malignant tumors in type 4; therefore, "type 3" most commonly refers to nonmalignant nonepithelial tumors, such as hemangioma. "Secondary tumors" refers to those that arise in surrounding tissues and invade the salivary gland, or those that metastasize to the salivary gland from distant sites.

Overall, this classification is much less relevant for prognostic and treatment purposes than the precise tumor type and the anatomic extent of tumor spread. For example, monomorphic adenoma and pleomorphic adenoma are both adenomas; however, monomorphic adenoma is unlikely to recur after enucleation, whereas pleomorphic adenoma frequently results in local recurrences, the need for multiple resections, and associated functional and cosmetic disability. Adenoid cystic carcinoma most commonly causes initial morbidity through permeation of surrounding tissues by means of perineural invasion, whereas other carcinomas are more likely to metastasize early in their course. The differing natural histories of individual tumor types thus must be taken into account during treatment planning. A critical factor in the prognosis and management of pleomorphic adenoma, carcinomas, and other malignancies is the involvement of the deep, superficial, or both portions of the parotid gland, the facial nerve, surrounding tissues, and metastatic sites.

Salivary Gland Tumor Staging

What It Classifies

The clinical stage of salivary gland tumors.

System

See Table 2-4.

References

O'Brien JC. Head and neck I: tumors. *Selected Readings in Plastic Surgery.* 1985;8(9).

Richards AM. The head and neck. In: Richards AM, ed. *Key Notes in Plastic Surgery.* Oxford: Blackwell Science Limited; 2002: 106-107.

Uses

Primary: Diagnosis, Treatment, Prognosis, Research

Secondary: Description

Limited/none: Etiology

Comments

Dr. Paul Oxley

All cancers with metastatic potential need to be defined using the TNM classification.

Table 2-4. Staging Salivary Gland Tumors

Stage I	T1a, N0, M0
	T2a, N0, M0
Stage II	T1b, N0, M0
	T2b, N0, M0
	T3a, N0, M0
Stage III	T3b, N0, M0
	T4a, N0, M0
	Any T (except T4b), N1, M0
Stage IV	T4b, Any N, M0
	Any T, N2 or 3, M0
	Any T, Any N, M1

Source: From "Head and neck I: tumors," O'Brien JC, *Selected Readings in Plastic Surgery*, 1995; 8(9). Copyright 1995 by *Selected Readings in Plastic Surgery.* Reprinted with permission.

Using this information, the stage of the tumor can be determined. Staging a tumor allows the treating physician to give a prognosis, as well as to determine which treatment options are available. Although often the main factor when determining treatment, many agencies also depend on patient age and comorbid conditions.

Staging is also useful to compare results among different treatment modalities and centers.

When learning this system it is more important to understand how the T, N, and M classifications are determined. The exact stage can be easily assessed from staging tables.

TNM Classification of Head and Neck Tumors

What It Classifies

Tumor characteristics with respect to depth of invasion and metastases.

System

See Table 2-5.

Table 2-5. Classification of Head and Neck Tumors

Primary Tumor (T): "a" signifies no local extension of tumor, "b" signifies local (nonmicroscopic) extension.

Tx	Primary tumor cannot be assessed			
T0	No evidence of primary tumor			
Tis	In situ primary			

	Lip, Oral Cavity	**Nasopharyngeal**	**Hypopharyngeal**	**Maxillary Sinus**
T1	<2 cm diameter	confined to one subsite	confined to one subsite	limited to antral mucosa
T2	2–4 cm diameter	more than one subsite	more than one subsite, no fixation	invades bone below Ohngren's line
T3	>4 cm diameter	extends beyond nasal cavity	invades larynx	invades bone above Ohngren's line
T4	invades adjacent structures	invades skull base or cranial nerves	invades neck soft tissue	invades into adjacent structures

Nodal Involvement (N):

Nx	Minimal requirements to assess nodes cannot be met
N0	No regional node involvement
N1	Single ipsilateral lymph node <3 cm in diameter
N2a	Single ipsilateral lymph node 3 to 6 cm in diameter
N2b	Multiple ipsilateral lymph nodes <6 cm in diameter
N2c	Bilateral or contralateral lymph nodes <6 cm in diameter
N3	Any neck with node >6 cm

Distant Metastases (M):

Mx	Minimal requirements to assess distant metastases cannot be met
M0	No distant metastases detected
M1	Distant metastases present

Source: From "Key notes in plastic surgery," Richards AM, ed, Blackwell Science Limited, 2002: 106–107. Copyright 2002 by Blackwell Publishing. Reprinted with permission.

References

O'Brien JC. Head and neck I: tumors. *Selected Readings in Plastic Surgery.* 1985;8(9).

Richards AM. The head and neck. In: Richards AM, ed. *Key Notes in Plastic Surgery.* Oxford: Blackwell Science Limited; 2002:106–107.

Uses

Primary: Diagnosis, Treatment, Research, Prognosis

Secondary: Description

Limited/none: Etiology

Comments

Dr. Paul Oxley

The evolution of clinical staging of cancer has made significant changes over the past 30 years. The American Joint Committee and the Union International Contra Cancer are the bodies that oversee the classification and staging of cancer. The TNM system is a standard used to describe most cancers. The system is designed to give a standard diagnosis for a given clinical presentation, as well as helping to direct treatment options based on relative prognosis.

Once the TNM classification has been determined, the staging of the cancer can be done, usually using a four-grade staging system. The higher the stage connotes a worsening prognosis.

Dr. Martin Jugenburg and Dr. Andrea Pusic

For a reconstructive surgeon, the value of any TNM and staging system lies in its ability to predict the extent of the defect, what subsequent treatment may follow (eg, radiation or chemotherapy) and prognosis. This, in return, allows the surgeon to plan his or her reconstructive strategy. As essential as the TNM stage information may be, it is still most important that the reconstructive surgeon maintains an open line of communication with the oncologic surgeon.

TNM Classification of Salivary Tumors

What It Classifies

Tumor characteristics with respect to depth of invasion and metastases.

System

See Table 2-6.

References

O'Brien JC. Head and neck I: tumors. *Selected Readings in Plastic Surgery.* 1985;8(9).

Richards AM. The head and neck. In: Richards AM, ed. *Key Notes in Plastic Surgery.* Oxford: Blackwell Science Limited; 2002: 106-107.

Table 2-6. TNM Classification of Salivary Gland Tumors

Primary Tumor (T): "a" signifies no local extension of tumor, "b" signifies local (non microscopic) extension.	
Tx	Primary tumor cannot be assessed
T0	No evidence of primary tumor
Tis	In situ primary
T1	<2 cm diameter in greatest dimension
T2	2 to 4 cm diameter in greatest dimension
T3	4 to 6 cm diameter in greatest dimension
T4	>6 cm in greatest dimension
Nodal Involvement (N):	
Nx	Minimal requirements to assess nodes cannot be met
N0	No regional node involvement
N1	Single ipsilateral lymph node <3 cm in diameter
N2a	Single ipsilateral lymph node 3 to 6 cm in diameter
N2b	Multiple ipsilateral lymph nodes <6 cm in diameter
N2c	Bilateral or contralateral lymph nodes <6 cm in diameter
N3	Any neck with node >6 cm
Distant Metastases (M):	
Mx	Minimal requirements to assess distant metastases cannot be met
M0	No distant metastases detected
M1	Distant metastases present

Uses

Primary: Description, Research, Diagnosis

Secondary: Treatment, Prognosis

Limited/none: Etiology

Comments

Dr. Paul Oxley

The evolution of clinical staging of cancer has made significant changes over the past 30 years. The American Joint Committee and the Union International Contra Cancer are the bodies that oversee the classification and staging of cancer. TNM is a standard system used to describe most cancers. The system is designed to give a standard diagnosis for a given clinical presentation, as well as help direct treatment options based on relative prognosis.

Once the TNM classification has been determined, the cancer is staged usually using a four point system. The higher the stage connotes a worsening prognosis.

Classifying salivary gland tumors can also be done using histologic features or the location of the primary. The histologic classification also includes nonmalignant tumors such as adenomas, which the TNM system does not.

Dr. Colleen McCarthy

Although the TNM staging system is useful in terms of predicting the extent of the defect, predicting disease recurrence and survival, and recommending oncologic treatment for patients with salivary gland tumors, this classification will have little other use for the reconstructive surgeon in planning their reconstruction. Immediately following salivary gland tumor resection, a plastic surgeon may be called upon to perform facial nerve grafts, create a soft tissue sling, and/or provide soft tissue for wound coverage.

Thus, following the surgical ablation of a salivary gland tumor, the reconstructive surgeon must assess both the volume and surface area requirements of the surgical defect, as well as the status of the facial nerve and its branches. A schema which further defines these postablative defects and their individual requirements, thereby facilitating surgical decision-making, is currently lacking.

Chapter 3
CONGENITAL

Cleft Lip Alveolus

What It Classifies

Different cleft patterns seen in the alveolus associated with cleft of the primary palate.

System

Type A: Narrow cleft, no collapse of alveolar arch

Type B: Narrow cleft, collapse of alveolar arch

Type C: Wide cleft, no collapse

Type D: Wide cleft, collapse

Reference

Byrd HS. Unilateral cleft lip. In: Aston SJ, Beasley RW, Thorne CHM, eds. *Grabb and Smith's Plastic Surgery*. 5th ed. Philadelphia, Pa: Lippincott-Raven Publishers; 1997:245.

Uses

Primary: Prognosis, Description

Secondary: Treatment, Diagnosis, Research

Limited/none: Etiology

Comments

Dr. Paul Oxley

This classification looks at the alveolus portion of the primary palate deformity. As the grade increases, the difficulty of surgical correction increases and the need for presurgical orthopedics increases. It does not describe the condition of the soft tissues, the extent of the palatal cleft, or what a wide versus narrow cleft is. In general, this is a reliable and easily applied classification. Most practitioners will use the descriptive form (eg, narrow, no collapse) rather than the letter type (eg, type A) when conveying clinical findings.

Dr. Cindy Verchere

I think this classification is mostly applicable at the time of bone graft planning. It may help to determine the severity of the cleft in order to recommend treatment and compare outcomes.

Tanzer Classification of Constricted Ear

What It Classifies

Severity of constricted (Tanzer Type IV A) ears.

System

Type I: Helical involvement only

Type IIA: Helix and scapha involved, no extra skin needed

Type IIB: Helix and scapha involved, extra skin needed

Type III: Extreme cupping deformity involving helix, scapha, antihelix and chonchal wall

Reference

Tanzer RC. The constricted (cup or lop) ear. *Plast Reconstr Surg.* 1975;55(4):406.

Uses

Primary: Diagnosis, Description

Secondary: Treatment, Prognosis, Research

Limited/none: Etiology

Comments

Dr. Paul Oxley

This classification is not as widely used as Tanzer's classification of auricular defects, and is more of a subclassification of that system. When people mention "Tanzer's classification" and don't specify which one, they are usually referring to the other.

This classification focuses on the more common constricted ear. It is a very precise system, leaving little space for subjective scoring in the case of 2A and 2B. Many treatment options exist for constricted ears, and having diagnosed the type, Tanzer offers corrections for each in his original paper. This degree of precision makes this a more useful classification in clinical practice and decision-making than the larger Tanzer classification, which has its primary use in research.

Some authors believe that type III should be viewed as a form of microtia and treated as such.

Dr. Doug Courtemanche

The practical application of this paper is that it guides the surgeon to a detailed assessment of the skin and cartilage deficiencies and deformities in three dimensions. The various treatment options mentioned and illustrated demonstrate that the problem needs to be considered in two parts. The first is the position, shape, size, and stability of the auricular framework and the second is the quality of the soft-tissue cover. Several procedures are described and referenced that are useful guides when planning correction of lop, cup, and constricted ears. I would agree that the more severe "tubular" ears are better thought of in the same way as "microtia" with a view to rib cartilage graft reconstruction being a better option for reconstruction.

Craniofacial Microsomia

What It Classifies

Clinical findings in the patient with hemifacial microsomia.

AKA

Harvold, Vargervik, and Chierici Classification

System

IA: The classic type characterized by unilateral facial underdevelopment without microphthalmos or ocular dermoids but with or without abnormalities of the vertebrae, heart, or kidneys

IB: Similar to type IA except for the presence of microphthalmos

IC: Bilateral asymmetric type in which one side is more severely involved.

ID: Complex type that does not fit the above but does not display limb deficiency, frontonasal phenotype, or ocular dermoids.

II: Limb deficiency type— unilateral or bilateral with or without ocular abnormalities.

III: Frontonasal type. Relative unilateral underdevelopment of the face in the presence of hypertelorism with or without ocular dermoids and vertebral, cardiac, or renal abnormalities.

IVA: Unilateral Goldenhar type with facial underdevelopment in association with ocular dermoids, with or without upper lid colobomas.

IVB: Bilateral form of IVA

References

Harvold EP, Vargervik K, Chierici G. *Treatment of Hemifacial Microsomia.* New York, NY: A.R. Liss; 1983.

McCarthy JG. Craniofacial microsomia. In: Aston SJ, Beasley RW, Thorne CHM, eds. *Grabb and Smith's Plastic Surgery.* 5th ed. Philadelphia, Pa: Lippincott-Raven Publishers; 1997:305.

Uses

Primary: Description, Diagnosis

Secondary: Etiology, Treatment

Limited/none: Research, Prognosis

Comments

Dr. Paul Oxley

One of many classification systems for hemifacial microsomia and the first widely published. It looks at the disorder from a clinical point of view, picking up major abnormalities but not really stratifying severity or separating the individual parts. As a result, two patients characterized by one subtype may have significantly different disease (Fig 3–1).

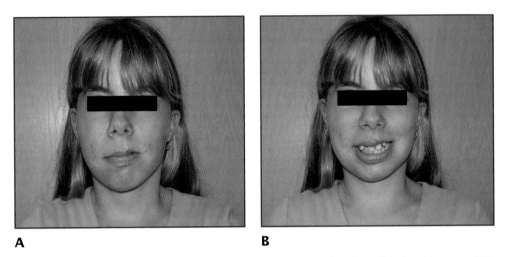

A

B

Fig 3-1. Hemifacial microsomia mouth with mouth closed (**A**) and open (**B**).

It has a limited role in research and is primarily a clinical tool for description of the condition. Prognosis is not correlated with progression through the classification. The Omens plus system is a better one for looking at the full breadth of the condition and is cited later in this chapter.

Encephaloceles

What It Classifies

Different types of herniation of cranial contents through abnormal openings in the bony structure of the central nervous system.

System

Encephaloceles are a collection of conditions of herniation of brain or lining through a defect in the cranium, usually in the midline. The defect may be a result of a craniofacial cleft.

1. Meningocele—meninges only

2. Meningoencephalocele—meninges and brain
3. Cystocele—meninges, brain, and ventricle
4. Myelocele—spinal cord

Reference

Hobar PC. Craniofacial anomalies II: syndromes and surgery. *Selected Readings in Plastic Surgery.* 1994;7(25):1.

Uses

Primary: Diagnosis

Secondary: Description, Treatment, Etiology

Limited/none: Prognosis, Research

Comments

Dr. Paul Oxley

This is an anatomic and pathologic classification of CNS herniation. It does not describe the location of the encephalocele and therefore modifiers are needed to fully describe the anomaly. In addition, it does not explain the cause or severity of the condition. The numeric classification is generally not used in communication, rather it is the specific name of the encephalocele.

This system is most useful as a learning tool to understand the different types of encephaloceles and what the differential diagnosis of one would be. Many conditions can lead to an encephalocele, and the treatment largely depends more on the cause than the anatomic constituents of the herniation.

Dr. Navraj Singh Heran

This system is simple, readily understood, readily taught, and just makes sense. One of the glaring omissions in the scale is the myelocystocele, a situation in which the spinal cord and cystic dilatation of the cord is herniated outward through the native site. It is a descriptive tool and not a scale at all.

Dr. Kevin L. Bush

Classification on the basis of the contents of the encephalocele is useful in determining what needs to be done with the contents themselves. However, with the exception of an inferior encephalocele, the vast majority of encephaloceles in the craniofacial skeleton contain non-functioning brain material and can essentially be amputated for the purposes of reconstruction. This particular classification is only useful for classifying the contents of the encephalocele but does not direct the physician toward the appropriate treatment required for those particular individuals with the condition.

Encephaloceles have many associated craniofacial distortions which are really as important or more important than the encephalocele itself. This classification does not take into account any of those abnormalities. It is not particularly useful in directing the treatment, research, or providing prognosis. It is only useful in directing the aspect of treatment that pertains to the possible resection of an encephalocele.

Frontoethmoidal Encephalomeningocele

What It Classifies

Locations and types of encephalomeningoceles affecting the frontal, orbital, and ethmoid regions of the skull.

System

See Table 3–1 and Figure 3–2.

Table 3–1. Frontoethmoidal Encephalomeningoceles

Types	Description
I	**Single external opening between frontal, nasal, ethmoidal, and orbital bones**
IA	Opening is limited between two bones of the area: Frontonasal Nasoethmoidal Naso-orbital
IB	Opening is extended transversely or cephalad to involve adjacent structures Frontonasal with orbital extension Frontonasal defect with bilateral extension to the orbit Frontonasal with cephalad extension Nasoethmoidal with orbital extension Nasoethmoidal with bilateral extension to the orbit Nasoethmoidal with cephalad extension
II	**Multiple external openings in the region**
IIA	All of the openings are limited types Naso-orbital type masses on each side One naso-orbital type mass and one nasoethmoidal type mass Naso-orbital type masses on each side and one nasoethmoidal type mass in the middle
IIB	One or more of the openings is/are extended type(s) that involve adjacent structures. One mass is type 1A naso-orbital and another is type IB nasoethmoidal with orbital extension Both masses are type IB nasoethmoidal with orbital extension

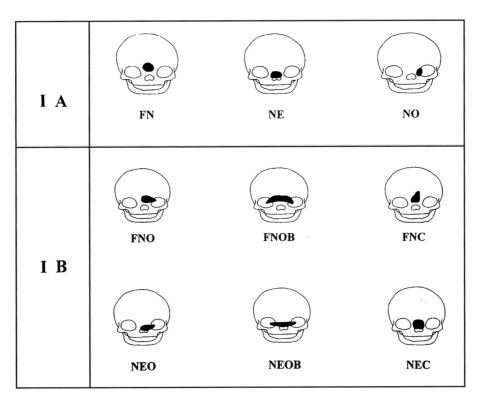

Fig 3–2. Frontoethmoidal encephalomeningoceles. Boonvisut et al. Morphologic study of 120 skull base defects in frontoethmoidal encephalomeningoceles. *Plast Reconstr Surg.* 1998;101(7):1784–1795. Copyright 1998 by Lippincott, Williams & Wilkins. Reprinted with permission.

Reference

Boonvisut S, Ladpli S, Sujatanond M, et al. Morphologic study of 120 skull base defects in frontoethmoidal encephalomeningoceles. *Plast Reconstr Surg.* 1998;101(7): 1784-1795.

Uses

Primary: Description, Diagnosis,

Secondary: Research, Etiology

Limited/none: Prognosis, Treatment

Comments

Dr. Paul Oxley

Herniation of the brain and meninges through a congenital defect in the cranium at the fusion of the frontal and ethmoidal bones is called frontoethmoidal encephalomeningocele. The treatment of these defects has generally been determined by which structures are involved. Most procedures now combine both an intracranial and extracranial approach so an understanding of the defect location is very important for proper operative planning.

In this study, 120 cases were reviewed and the craniual defects studied including CT scans and intraoperative findings. The authors found more types of defects than had previously been reported in other studies. From this they devised the above classification system. It is useful in describing the pathway of herniation and combining those with certain common characteristics.

As many procedures are based on the same approach, this classification does not direct the type of therapy for each specific type. In addition, as there are so many subtypes for each type that have not been given a specific number, the word for word anatomic description still needs to be given and recorded each time.

Dr. Navraj Singh Heran

The basic rules of a scale or scoring system is that it should be simple, intuitive, and reproducible. This scale meets neither of the first two criteria and, as a result, is not easily reproducible. Unfortunately, the diseases in this group have specific treatment implications as well as natural history implications and that is why a scale is valuable. Unfortuanately, this scale is just as complex as the encephaloceles that need to be classified.

The pictorial representation is also not very helpful. Some things just cannot be classified too readily and broader categories may be better. I just would not know how to do it for this disease and have it make any clinical impact.

Dr. Doug Courtemanche

This is a detailed and elaborate classification scheme of the bony defect in fronto-orbitalethmoidal encephaloceles.

The scheme does not discuss the soft tissue problems associated with the deformities except to document the frequency of lachrymal duct abnormalities. The comments related to the malposition of the medial orbital wall in these defects without true hypertelorism are important in understanding the dysmorphology.

The use of detailed physical examination and detailed 3-D CT study would be considered essential and the standard of care for diagnosis and treatment planning for patients with this deformity.

Hemifacial Microsomia—Ear Anomalies

What It Classifies

Ear anomalies in hemifacial microsomia.

AKA

Meurman Classification.

System

Type 1: All components present but hypoplastic, malformed

Type 2: Atresia of external auditory meatus with vertical remnant of skin and cartilage

Type 3: Complete absence of all structures ± small lobule

References

McCarthy JG. Craniofacial microsomia. In: Aston SJ, Beasley RW, Thorne CHM, eds. *Grabb and Smith's Plastic Surgery.* 5th ed. Philadelphia, Pa: Lippincott-Raven Publishers; 1997:305.

Meurman Y. Congenital microtia and meatal atresia. *Arch Otolaryngol.* 1957;66:443.

Uses

Primary: Diagnosis, Description

Secondary: Treatment, Research

Limited/none: Prognosis, Etiology

Comments

Dr. Paul Oxley

Hemifacial microsomia is composed of deformities that often have their own variations that often do not correspond to attempts at classification. Mandibular hypoplasia and auricular hypoplasia may be present in varying degrees independent of each other, necessitating different classifications to best describe each area of concern. Unfortunately, this makes classification of hemifacial microsomia somewhat cumbersome.

The above system looks specifically at auricular hypoplasia and breaks it down into three large groups of clinical significance more than descriptive precision. Treatment is largely directed by degree of hypoplasia or aplasia, but can be influenced by a surgeon's preference, the status of the contralateral ear, and comorbid conditions. There is debate whether hearing in the affected ear is correlated with the severity of the deformity.

Dr. Gordon Wilkes

I do not find this classification of ear deformities particularly useful. It is very general. Grade 2 is basically a lobule type microtia with or without an external auditory canal (Tanzer 2a or 2b). Grade 3 varies from anotia to an atypical lobule type microtia. The Meurman system is likely of some benefit in helping categorize the patients more effectively if used in conjunction with the Pruzansky system for long-term follow-up. For treatment planning of ear reconstruction in Cranio-facial Microsomia, however, other classification systems are more beneficial.

Mandibular Deformity in Hemifacial Microsomia

What It Classifies

Degree of mandibular hypoplasia in hemifacial microsomia.

AKA

Pruzansky Classification, Mulliken-Kaban Classification

System

Type I: Mild mandibular ramus hypoplasia. The body is minimally affected

Type IIa: Severe mandibular hypoplasia with functional TMJ present.

- Condyle and ramus are small
- Head of condyle flattened

Type IIb: Severe mandibular hypoplasia with nonarticulating TMJ.

- Glenoid fossa absent
- Condyle hinged on a flat/convex infratemporal surface.

Type III: Aplasia of the mandibular ramus and therefore absent TMJ.

References

Kaban LB, Moses MH, Mulliken JB. Surgical correction of hemifacial microsomia in the growing child. *Plast Reconstr Surg.* 1988;82:979.

McCarthy JG. Craniofacial microsomia. In: Aston SJ, Beasley RW, Thorne CHM, eds. *Grabb and Smith's Plastic Surgery.* 5th ed. Philadelphia, Pa: Lippincott-Raven Publishers; 1997:305.

Mulliken JB, Kaban LB. Analysis and treatment of hemifacial microsomia in childhood. *Clin Plast Surg.* 1987;14:91.

Pruzansky S. Not all dwarfed mandibles are alike. *Birth Defects.* 1969;5:120.

Uses

Primary: Description, Diagnosis

Secondary: Treatment, Prognosis, Research

Limited/none: Etiology

Comments

Dr. Paul Oxley

The original classification by Pruzansky (1969) included three mandibular types (I, II, and III) and did not divide type II. It used the mandible and TMJ as the center of reference. It was modified by Mulliken and Kaban in 1987 to denote the existence of a functional TMJ (type IIa) and a useless glenoid fossa and TMJ (type IIb). This distinction between types IIa and IIb has important implications for operative planning and prognosis.

This is a very useful and very succinct classification of mandibular hypoplasia in the diagnosis of hemifacial microsomia. Though there is a little room for interpretation between types I and IIa, there is very clear distinction between the other groups. Therefore, it is very useful as a descriptive tool and to convey diagnosis. Treatment and prognosis depend largely on the group, as well as comorbid conditions and time (age) at treatment.

Dr. Gordon Wilkes

This classification system describes only the mandibular deformity associated with craniofacial microsomia. It effectively categorizes the deformity into increasing degrees of severity. This is useful from both a treatment and prognostic point of view. This classification system is also beneficial in the era of evidence-based medicine as reference points for comparing reconstructive results using different treatment approaches. This is the mark of a useful classification system. Although there is a degree of correlation between the degree of mandibular deformity and other associated deformities (soft tissue, auricular, nerve, and maxilla) in craniofacial microsomia, this classification system does not address this. As a result, other authors (Edgerton and Marsh, Tenconi and Hall, Munro and Lauritzen, David and Vento, La Brie, and Mulliken) have presented other classification systems to try to encompass all the anatomic variations associated with craniofacial microsomia. The challenge is to find a system simple enough yet comprehensive enough to have practical value for classification, treatment planning, and analysis of outcomes.

Hemifacial Microsomia—Multisystem

What It Classifies

Combines three systems for grading severity of hemifacial microsomia.

AKA

SAT Classification

System

S: Skeletal deformity (based on Pruzansky)
- 0. None
- 1. Mandibular hypoplasia
- 2. Severe mandibular hypoplasia, Limited/no TMJ
- 3. Mandibular aplasia
- 4. Orbital involvement
- 5. Orbital dystopia

A: Auricular deformity (based on Meurman)
- 0. None
- 1. Auricular hypoplasia, all structures present
- 2. Vertical remnant of skin and cartilage present, meatal atresia
- 3. Total auricular aplasia

T: Soft tissue deficiency
- 0. None
- 1. Mild
- 2. Moderate
- 3. Severe

Reference

David DJ, Mahatumarat C, Cooter RD. Hemifacial microsomia: a multisystem classification. *Plast Reconstr Surg.* 1987;80:525.

Uses

Primary: Diagnosis, Description

Secondary: Treatment, Research

Limited/none: Prognosis, Etiology

Comments

Dr. Paul Oxley

This classification tries to combine the elements of the Pruzansky classification and the Meurman classification to give a single score for patients with hemifacial microsomia. It adds the soft tissue defect element not seen in the other classifications.

The classification itself is presented in the same manner that cancers are presented using a TNM score. For example, a patient can be S3 A1 T2.

As this system gives a view to more than one system, it provides a greater picture of the patient's condition than the other systems. As it relies on those systems it takes advantage of their strengths. It leaves out some of the specific findings categorized in the Munro classification.

The SAT system helps the clinician look at each patient as a whole and provides a framework form which to treat the whole patient and plan staged, complementary procedures

Dr. Cindy Verchere

I think this a good working classification system providing a generally logical progression of severity, and its relation to the TNM classification makes it familiar.

There are, in my opinion, some flaws in that the "soft tissue" descriptions are very subjective, and the mandibular and orbital involvements are not necessarily so easily separated or sequential: you may have to choose a number which describes the more clinically important deformity, even if both are involved. These subjective decisions may affect interrater reliability.

Unilateral Craniofacial Microsomia

What It Classifies

Clinical findings in hemifacial microsomia.

AKA

Munro and Lauritzen Classification

System

IA: The craniofacial skeleton is only mildly hypoplastic and the occlusal plane is horizontal.

IB: The skeleton is as in IA but the occlusal plane is canted.

II: The condyle and part of the affected ramus are absent

III: In addition to the findings in type II, the zygomatic arch and glenoid fossa are absent

IV: Uncommon type with hypoplasia of the zygoma and medial and posterior displacement of the lateral orbital wall

V: The most extreme type with inferior displacement of the orbit with a decrease in orbital volume.

References

Lauritzen CG, Munro IR, Ross RB. Classification and treatment of hemifacial microsomia. *Scand J Plast Reconstr Surg.* 1985; 19:33.

McCarthy JG. Craniofacial microsomia. In: Aston SJ, Beasley RW, Thorne CHM, eds. *Grabb and Smith's Plastic Surgery.* 5th ed. Philadelphia, Pa: Lippincott-Raven Publishers; 1997:305.

Munro IR. One-stage reconstruction of the temporomandibular joint in hemifacial microsomia. *Plast Reconstr Surg.* 1980; 66:699.

Munro IR, Lauritzen CG, Classifcation and treatment of hemifacial microsomia. In: Caronni EP, ed. *Craniofacial Surgery.* Boston, Mass: Little, Brown & Co; 1985:391–400.

Uses

Primary: Description, Diagnosis, Treatment

Secondary: Research, Prognosis

Limited/none: Etiology

Comments

Dr. Paul Oxley

This classification followed that of Harvold and colleagues and focused on surgical planning for correction of the condition. It looks at the clinical aspects of the dis-order, focusing on the skeleton. It is useful in determining which problems can be addressed surgically.

As it is primarily a clinical tool, it has limited use in research. It does not subdivide all categories, nor does it describe severity of any given problem, often commenting only on the presence of the problem.

OMENS-Plus

What It Classifies

Anomalies associated with hemifacial microsomia.

AKA

OMENS

System

Orbital classes

O0: Normal orbital size and position

O1: Abnormal orbital size

O2: Abnormal orbital position

O3: Abnormal orbital size and position

Mandibular classes

M0: Normal mandible

M1: Mandible and glenoid fossa are small with a short ramus

M2: The mandible ramus is short and abnormally shaped

M2a: Glenoid fossa in anatomically acceptable position in relation to opposite TMJ

M2b: TMJ inferiorly, medially, and anteriorly displaced with hypo-plastic condyle

M3: Complete absence of ramus, glenoid fossa, and TMJ

External ear anomaly classes

E0: Normal ear

E1: Mild hypoplasia and cupping with al structures present

E2: Absence of external auditory canal with variable hypoplasia of the concha

E3: Malpositioned lobule with absence of auricle

Facial nerve classes
(Other cranial nerves can be graded as well, for example N10 or N9)

N70: No facial nerve involvement

N71: Upper facial nerve involvement (temporal and zygomatic branches

N72: Lower facial nerve involvement (buccal, mandibular, and cervical branches

N73: All branches of facial nerve affected

Soft tissue deficiency classes

S0: No obvious soft tissue or muscle deficiency

S1: Minimal subcuateous/muscle deficiency

S2: Moderate deficiency

S3: Sever soft tissue deficiency caused by subcutaneous and muscular hypoplasia

OMENS-plus

Any associated extracranial anomaly

References

Vento RA, LaBrie RA, Mulliken JB. The OMENS classification of hemifacial microsomia. *Cleft Palate Craniofac J.* 1991;28:68.

Cohen SR, Levitt CA, Simms C, Burstein FD. Airway disorders in hemifacial microsomia. *Plast Reconstr Surg.* 1999;103(1):27–33.

Cousley RRJ. A comparison of two classification systems for hemifacial microsomia, *Brit J Oral Maxillofac Surg.* 1993;31:78.

Note. Portions of this section were taken from "OMENS-Plus: analysis of craniofacial and extracraniofacial anomalies in hemifacial microsomia," Horgan JE, Padwa BL, LaBrie RA, Mulliken JB, *Cleft Palate Craniofac J.* 1995;32:405. Copyright 1995 by Allen Press Publishing Services. Reprinted with permission.

Uses

Primary: Description, Diagnosis, Research

Secondary: Treatment, Prognosis

Limited/none: Etiology

Comments

Dr. Paul Oxley

Hemifacial microsomia is a complex facial disorder affecting many tissues resulting in one side of the face being smaller than the other. It is usually a unilateral anomaly, but quite fequently it can be a bilateral. The severity and complexity varies dramatically, and can also be associated with extracranial anomalies including cardiac, skeletal, renal, and CNS findings.

The OMENS classification was designed by Vento et al to describe and grade the five major craniofacial anomalies seen in hemifacial microsomia. They recognized the mandibular involvement as the cornerstone of the disorder. The original classification called for four classes of severity within each anatomic location, with 0 being normal and 3 being the most severe. It allowed for bilateral disease in that each side is described separately in each category. Subcategories exist in some cases. The OMENS-plus category was later added by Horgan et al to describe patients who also have extracranial anomalies.

This system is very concise and easy to use. Except for the soft tissue scoring and relatively vague minimum criteria, the scores are objective with little room for individual interpretation. The system is useful for comparing a rare disease between sites and facilitating treatment and research. From the list of scores, a surgeon could describe operative options for most patients. Different treatment options exist for each level of severity, though with this system a surgeon can plan complementary procedures to minimize operative time and to optimize end results.

In 1993, Cousley compared the OMENS classification to the SAT system and found the former to be more comprehensive and useful.

Hypertelorism (Munro)

What It Classifies

Medial orbital wall shape in hypertelorism.

System

A: Parallel medial walls, widened

B: Lateral bulge in medial walls at anterior portion only

C: Lateral bulge in medial walls at mid portion

D: Lateral bulge in medial walls at posterior portion (Fig 3-3)

Reference

Munro IR, Das SK. Improving results in orbital hypertelorism correction. *Ann Plast Surg.* 1979;2:499–507.

Uses

Primary: Treatment, Description, Etiology

Secondary: Prognosis, Diagnosis, Research

Limited/none:

Comments

Dr. Paul Oxley

This classification defines the shape of the ethmoid and medial orbital wall in the patient with congenital hypertelorism. It does not specifically comment on the severity of the hypertelorism, which is based on the distance between the orbits and is measured as the intraorbital distance (IOD). Tessier used the IOD as the basis for his classification. Rather, the Munro scheme categorizes the condition by the effect the underlying cause (eg, cleft) has on the bony structures confined between the orbits.

Congenital hypertelorism has many causes, including craniosynostosis, encephalocele, or facial cleft. Again, this classification does not address etiology. It simply describes the interorbital deformity and suggests how it might be surgically corrected.

Both etiology and severity are important when determining prognosis and treatment options. Diagnosis with this system requires radiologic imaging (CT scan) to best define the condition prior to surgery. Unlike many classifications that are either clinical or research oriented, this one applies to both aspects.

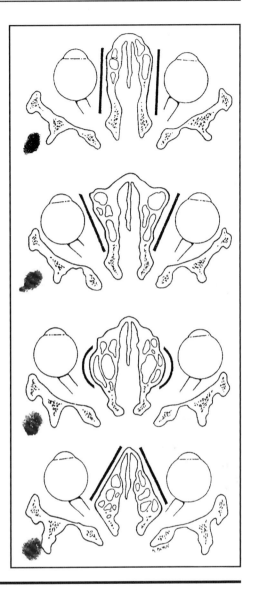

Fig 3–3. Hypertelorism, Munro IR, Das SK. Improving results in orbital hypertelorism correction. *Ann Plast Surg.* 1979;2:499–507. Copyright 1979 by Lippincott, Williams & Wilkins. Reprinted with permission.

Dr. Kevin L. Bush

The most commonly used classification for hypertelorism is, in fact, classifying the severity of hypertelorism on the basis of intraorbital distance. The advantage of Munro's classification is that it provides more information which is important in the surgical management of hypertelorism as it directs the surgeon toward areas which may need to be addressed at the time of surgery.

However, the classification does not provide the surgeon with an easily measurable external means of classifying hypertelorism which may direct the surgeon toward making the decision whether surgery is required. Its second problem is that is also requires a CT scan in order to apply the classification.

Hypertelorism

What It Classifies

Diagnostic categories of hypertelorism based on anatomic and morphogenetic classifications.

System

1. Frontonasal malformation: Hypertelorism and broadened nasal root with:
   A. Median nasal groove with bifid tip
   B. Minor: Deep median facial groove
   B. Major: True clefting of the nose or both nose and upper lip or palate
   C. Unilateral or bilateral notching of the ala nasi
   D. Combination of B Major and C
2. Craniofrontonasal dysplasia
3. Craniofacial cleft(s)
4. Encephalocele
5. Miscellaneous group
   Chromosomal
   Syndromic disorders.

Reference

Tan ST, Mulliken JB. Hypertelorism: nosologic analysis of 90 patients. *Plast Reconstr Surg.* 1997;99(2):317–327.

Uses

Primary: Etiology, Description, Diagnosis, Research

Secondary: Treatment

Limited/none: Prognosis

Comments

Dr. Paul Oxley

Hypertelorism is the condition where the intraorbital distance is greater than normal. It is not a diagnosis, rather it is a physical finding in many different craniofacial anomalies. Because different etiologies can result in the same appearance, understanding or attempting to define hypertelorism can be challenging. The key issue is not only to determine that hypertelorism exists but whether it is caused by pathology related to the orbits themselves or the space between the orbits. Once true hypertelorism has been determined, to which category does it belong?

This classification attempts and succeeds in combining the anatomic and morphogenetic classifications of hypertelorism. Although the anatomic scheme addresses the physical characteristics (eg, absolute distance between orbits, orbital vs interorbital), the dysmorphogenetic aspect suggests pathogenesis. Better understanding of the basis for the hypertelorism better allows the surgeon to decide on the correct management.

Surgical management depends on both the cause and the severity. Different surgical approaches are used for interorbital versus orbital hypertelorism and the different causes of each.

Hypertelorism (Tessier)

What It Classifies

Width or severity of hypertelorism based on intraorbital distance (IOD).

AKA

Günther-Tessier grading system of hypertelorism

System

See Table 3-2.

References

Tan ST, Mulliken JB. Hypertelorism: nosologic analysis of 90 patients. *Plast Reconstr Surg.* 1997;99(2):317-327.

Tessier P. Experiences in the treatment of orbital hypertelorism. *Plast Reconstr Surg.* 1974;53:1.

Table 3-2. Günther-Tessier Grading System of Hypertelorism

Degree	Description
1	IOD 30–34 mm
2	IOD of 35–39 mm, with normal orientation and shape of the orbits
3	IOD >40 mm, with defects in the cribriform plate, orbital region, and lateral canthus

IOD = Interocular distance.

Uses

Primary: Research, Description, Diagnosis

Secondary: Treatment, Prognosis

Limited/none: Etiology

Comments

Dr. Paul Oxley

Tessier's classification, or severity rating, of hypertelorism relies on measurement between the dacryon or anterior lacrimal crest of one orbit to the other. The measurement is not made by interpupillary distance as the globe itself may be abnormally rotated or divergent strabismus may be present. Also, intercanthal distance can be exaggerated by excess soft tissue or traumatic telecanthus. This system assumes that the hypertelorism is symmetric, in so much that both orbits are displaced equally from the midline (Fig 3-4).

The grading is based purely on distance as measured in a radiograph. The normal values for hypertelorism increase with age and reach adult range around 12 years of age. This system focuses on the adult norms. Tan and Mulliken used standard deviation from the age and gender matched norms to define hypertelorism, thus adapting this system to younger patients. They suggested the following:

First degree: interorbital distance 2 to 4 SD greater than the normal mean

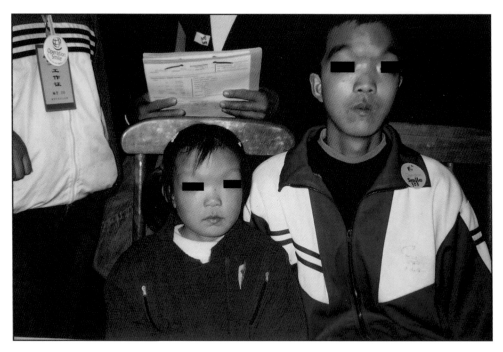

Fig 3–4. Hypertelorism in siblings.

Second degree: interorbital distance 4.1 to 8 SD greater than the normal mean

Third degree: interorbital distance more than 8 SDs greater than the normal mean

Neither the original or modified approach takes into account the cause of the hypertelorism which generally dictates treatment and prognosis.

Kernahan Striped-Y

What It Classifies

Cleft lip and palate.

System

See Figure 3-5.

References

Kernahan DA, Stark RB. A new classification for cleft lip and cleft palate. *Plast Reconstr Surg.* 1958;22:435.

Kernahan DA. The striped Y: a symbolic classification of cleft lips and palates. *Plast Reconstr Surg.* 1971;47:469.

Smith AW, Khoo AK, Jackson IT. A modification of the Kernahan "Y" classification in cleft lip and palate deformities. *Plast Reconstr Surg.* 1998:102(6):1842–1847.

Uses

Primary: Description, Diagnosis

Secondary: Research, Treatment, Prognosis

Limited/none: Etiology

Comments

Dr. Paul Oxley

Cleft lip and palate can be described by the extent of the defect and the affected tissues; however, it is difficult to convey this in a simple form. Kernahan introduced the striped-Y as a way to easily record

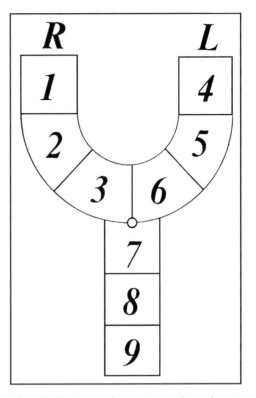

Fig 3–5. Kernahan striped-Y classification. Smith AW. *Plast Reconstr Surg.* 1998;102(6):1842–1847. Copyright 1998 by Lippincott, Williams & Wilkins. Reprinted with permission.

not only the location of the cleft but also whether it is complete or incomplete. Each number represents an anatomic location on the lip and palate:

One and 4 are lip, 2 and 5 alveolus, 3 and 6 hard palate extending to the incisive foramen (which is expressed as the small circle at the center of the Y), 7 and 8 are portions of the hard palate, and 9 the soft palate.

The description of a cleft can then be expressed either using the diagram itself by shading in the affected areas, or the numbers assigned to each area. For example, complete cleft on the right would be 123789. Partially cleft structures could be partially shaded in the diagram, but not easily expressed numerically. The picture (Fig 3–6) would be identified by shading all areas on the Y.

Kernahan's striped-Y conveys diagnosis and treatment options, although many exist for each problem. It is somewhat useful in research as it simplifies the expression of the problem and allows easy comparison between clefts, but as a visual map of a cleft it is difficult to transfer to a spread sheet.

This system does not easily represent a microform cleft, a small band (Simonart's band), the location of the cleft palate relative to the vomer, or the degree of cleft nasal deformity. Several attempts have been made to modify Kernahan's original scheme, including different ways of shading the diagram or adding extra parts to the Y. For example, hatch marks can be used to describe a submucous cleft. Modifications of the original have been done by Millard and Jackson to include nasal floor and alar rim clefting. A recent alphanumeric modification by Smith and Khoo (see next section) helps facilitate the expression of key components of the cleft and placement of that information onto a spread sheet.

Dr. Gordon Wilkes

Historically describing a cleft in an easy, yet comprehensive format has been a challenge. Pure descriptive terms are cumbersome and time consuming. Record keeping needs to be accurate but efficient when used in a busy clinical environment. The Kernahan classification went a long way to solving many of the problems of recording clefts in a logical straightforward manner. Although not perfect, it serves as the basis for other attempts to improve this classification system. The numerical system lends itself for ease of database collection of cleft data. The easily understandable visual appearance of the system on a chart allows for easy description of the problem to others. It makes teaching health care providers at all levels relatively straightforward. The continued use of the Kernahan classification system although not perfect, demonstrates a general feeling that it is the best system currently available. Suggestions for improvement one hopes will further improve it. The challenge is to improve the system but maintain its inherent simplicity.

Dr. Cindy Verchere

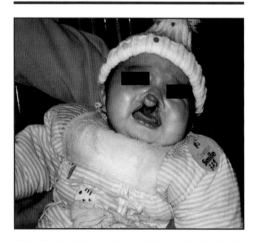

Fig 3–6. Complete bilateral cleft lip and palate.

The beauty of the original Kernahan-Y was in its simple visual description of a cleft. I rarely use the numbers clinically. It is easily drawn and filled in for most clefts, and looking at it allows the reader to know immediately what the actual cleft might look like. Modifying this classification, as by Smith and Khoo, may allow a more standardized job of describing Simonart's bands and submucous clefts, but some of the subtle shading possible in the original Y is lost.

Modified Kernahan Striped-Y

What It Classifies

Cleft lip and palate.

System

1. All right-sided clefts are designated by numerals without prime and left-sided clefts by numerals that are primed. For example, 1 means a complete right cleft lip and 1' means a complete left cleft lip (Fig 3–7).
2. Incomplete cleft lips vary from microform to one-third to two-thirds, and these are classified as *a-c* and *a'-c'* for right and left, respectively. Lips with Simonart's band are classified as *d*.
3. The alveolus is documented as 2 or 2'. No allowance is made for minor degrees of clefting of the alveolus, as this has little bearing on management.
4. The palate anterior to the incisive foramen and posterior to the alveolus is documented as 3 or 3'.
5. The secondary palate, lying posterior to the incisive foramen, is subdivided into three segments based on the anatomic segments involved in the cleft: 4 denotes a cleft up to the palatine process of the maxillary bone; 5 is a cleft up to the palatine process of the palatine bone; 6 is a cleft including the soft palate only; and the letter a denotes a submucous cleft.

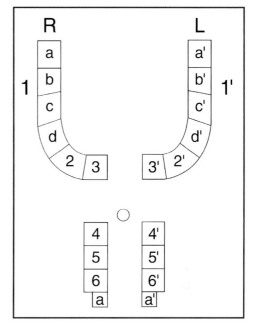

Fig 3–7. Modified Kernahan striped-Y. Smith AW. *Plast Reconstr Surg.* 1998; 102(6):1842–1847. Copyright 1998 by Lippincott, Williams & Wilkins. Reprinted with permission.

Reference

Smith AW, Khoo AK, Jackson IT. A modification of the Kernahan "Y" classification in cleft lip and palate deformities. *Plast Reconstr Surg.* 1998;102(6):1842–1847.

Uses

Primary: Description, Diagnosis, Research

Secondary: Treatment, Prognosis

Limited/none: Etiology

Comments

Dr. Paul Oxley

Kernahan's original striped-Y was a breakthrough in cleft lip and palate classification as it simplified the expression of the cleft. Its shortfallings, however, have led to many modifications.

This system gives an alphanumeric representation of each cleft. It encompasses different forms including microform clefts, soft tissue bands, and occult clefts. The right and left are differentiated by placing a prime next to a number for left-sided clefts. It also helps express the relationship of the cleft palate versus the vomer. The first number indicates where a cleft starts and the second number where it ends. For a cleft with only one side, the unaffected side is expressed as 00. For example, a complete left-sided cleft would be 00/1'6'.

The system does not attempt to include information about the cleft lip nasal deformity, velopharynx, or premaxilla. It focuses solely on the cleft lip and palate, and can just as easily describe complex clefts as well as simple ones. The study by Smith et al showed that this system is easily learned and applied by medical students as well as staff. It does not directly propose treatment as there are multiple surgical options for a given cleft, though the use of the system would allow a surgeon who has never seen the patient to plan the repair.

Dr. Cindy Verchere

The beauty of the original Kernahan-Y was in its simple visual description of a cleft. I rarely used the numbers clinically. It was easily drawn and filled in for most clefts, and looking at it allowed the reader to know immediately what the actual cleft might look like. I think numerically renaming the stripes is more of a research tool "improvement" than clinical improvement. To use clinically, one has to change the numbers and primes back into stripes and sides to "see" the cleft. This modified classification does a more standardized job of describing Simonart's bands and submucous clefts, but some of the subtle shading possible in the original Y is lost.

Congenital Nasal Anomalies

What It Classifies

Different types of congenital defects affecting the nose.

System

See Table 3–3

Table 3–3. Congenital Nasal Anomalies

Type	Description
I	***Hypoplasia and Atrophy***
	Agenesis of parts
	Arhinia—complete or partial
	Cartilage
	Bone
	Columella
	Hypoplasia of parts
	Heminose
	Nostril stenosis
	Piriform aperture stenosis
	Choanal atresia
	Nasal hypoplasia
	Craniofacial Syndromes
	Craniosynostosis
	Craniofacial dysostosis
	Binder
	Hemifacail microsomia
	Facial nerve palsy
	Hunermann
	Treacher Collins
	Byrne
	Fraser
	Trichorhinophalangeal
	Delleman

continues

Table 3–3. *continued*

Type	Description
II	***Hyperplasia and Duplications***
	Multiple or parts
	Proboscis
	Nostrils
	Columella
	Hemifacial hypertrophy
	Hyperplasia of tissues
III	***Atypical Clefts***
	Tessier 0/14
	Frontonasal dysplasia, median facial cleft
	Craniofrontonasal dysplasia
	Frontonasal encephalocele
	Tessier 1/13
	Tessier 2/12
	Tessier 3/13
	Cleft lip nasal deformity
IV	***Neoplasms and Vascular Anomalies***
	Benign lesions
	Hairy nevus
	Glioma
	Dermoid
	Pilomatrixoma
	Neurofibroma
	Sinus tract
	Polyp/nostril plug
	Lipoma
	Malignant lesions
	Vascular anomalies
	Vascular malformations
	Hemangiomas

Reference

Losee JE, Kirschner RE, Whitaker LA, Bartlett SP. Congenital nasal anomalies: a classification scheme. *Plast Reconstr Surg.* 2004; 113(2):676–689.

Uses

Primary: Research, Diagnosis, Etiology

Secondary: Description

Limited/none: Treatment, Prognosis

Comments

Dr. Paul Oxley

Nasal anomalies have many different types of presentation, from aplasia to duplication and clefts to neoplasms (Fig 3-8). This classification looked at developing simple morphogenic categories for nasal anomalies using a database of over 260 patients.

This is a very comprehensive categorization of nasal anomalies. It is useful to the student as a framework from which to learn nasal anomalies and how they

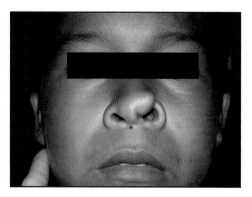

Fig 3–8. Nasal cleft.

relate to others. It requires further knowledge to understand each anomaly. Treatment options vary significantly and are not natural extensions of this classification system. It is useful in research for looking at the prevalence of different types and in trying to determine etiology.

Dr. Cindy Verchere

This is a very comprehensive classification and would not likely be very useful on a day-to-day basis, except to perhaps create complete differential diagnoses. It would be helpful to prepare papers, talks, photo filing, or study schedules to ensure a complete representation of anomalies, much like the IFSSH hand anomaly classification can be used.

Orbitotemporal Neurofibromatosis

What It Classifies

Extent of orbital involvement in cases of neurofibromatosis and the functional ability of the eye.

System

See Table 3–4.

References

Hobar PC. Craniofacial anomalies II: syndromes and surgery. *Selected Readings in Plastic Surgery.* 1994;7(25):1.

Jackson IT, Carbonnel A, Potparic Z, Shaw K. Orbitotemporal neurofibromatosis: classification and treatment. *Plast Reconstr Surg.* 1993;92(1):1–11.

Uses

Primary: Description, Diagnosis, Treatment

Secondary: Etiology, Research, Prognosis

Limited/none:

Comments

Dr. Paul Oxley

This classification was designed to describe and direct treatment in cases of neurofibromatosis affecting the orbit. The authors recognized that this condition, although benign in nature, can cause significant functional and cosmetic problems.

The condition is broken down into the three categories seen above. There is no clear distinction between types 1 and 2 with respect to the soft tissue involvement; however, type 2 does indicate the bone changes secondary to the condition. As some boney or soft tissue changes may be minor, this system is somewhat open to individual interpretation. The biggest problem is deciding what constitutes significant bony involvement. As for placing patients into group 3, this is easier, though with very young children this can be difficult to measure.

For these reasons, this system is more valuable as a clinical tool than a research tool. That is, it lacks the precision needed in a research tool. Otherwise the categories clearly describe the basic problem and the authors offer surgical options for each of these groups in the original articles.

Table 3–4. Orbitotemporal Neurofibromatosis

Category	Description
1	Orbital soft tissue involvement with a seeing eye.
2	Orbital soft tissue and significant bony involvement with a seeing eye.
3	Orbital soft tissue and significant bony involvement with a blind or absent eye.

Dr. Kevin L. Bush

Neurofibromatosis is indeed a difficult condition. Classifications in this particular region of the facial skeleton which is involved with neurofibromatosis need to clearly delineate the involvement of the eye. From a practical point of view radical dissection of and removal of soft tissue in the orbit is often significantly limited by the involvement of the seeing eye.

The second part of any assessment of neurofibromatosis in this particular region has to do with whether there is significant bony involvement especially at the orbital apex. The more severe the condition (ie, a nonseeing eye with bony involvement at the orbital apex) the easier the algorithm for treatment becomes simply because the risk of loss of vision is no longer part of the equation. This particular classification clearly delineates that limiting factor for surgical treatment in orbital temporal neurofibromatosis. This is a good classification for clinical use.

Plagiocephaly

What It Classifies

The causes of frontal plagiocephaly.

System

See Table 3–5.

Reference

Glat PM, Freund RM, Spector JA, et al. A classification of plagiocephaly utilizing a three-dimensional computer analysis of cranial base landmarks. *Ann Plast Surg.* 1996; 36(5):469–474.

Uses

Primary: Description, Diagnosis, Etiology

Secondary: Treatment, Research

Limited/none: Prognosis

Comments

Dr. Paul Oxley

The diagnosis of plagiocephaly has been classified previously by Bruneteau and Mulliken in 1992. The purpose of this classification system is to categorize patients and to assist in treatment planning. They described three types of frontal plagiocephaly: synostotic, compensational, and deformational.

Table 3–5. Plagiocephaly

Type	Description
I	Resulting from cranial suture synostosis
II	Nonsynostotic etiology
III	Associated with craniofacial microsomia

The above classification was designed to develop a simple system based on the earlier one of Mulliken and Bruneteau. Preoperative CT scans were used as the basis of this classification. Nine lateral landmarks from each side and two midline landmarks were used to determine extent and effect of the synostosis. The authors determined three major types of frontal plagiocephaly as shown in their classification system. By using CT scans with multiple points, they are able to show both vertical and horizontal growth arrest.

The authors recognize that given the small number of patients used to determine this system (30), it may need future refining to be applicable in preoperative diagnosis and treatment planning.

Dr. Navraj Singh Heran

This system is not commonly used among neurosurgeons in the field of pediatrics as far as I am aware. During training I did not study or utilize this system and none of the neurosurgeons I worked with use the system. The rationale is quite simple: either there is a problem with a suture resulting in differential cranial growth (type I), or there is an external influence, such as the child's position during upbringing that results in "positional" plagiocephaly (type II). The type III variety, one in which the head is small, is extremely uncommon and generally related to craniofacial syndromic situations such as Crouzon, Apert, or Pfeiffer syndromes. This latter type is extremely characteristic as an abnormality, and unlikely to be confused with the two former varieties by medical practitioners in general, let alone pediatric neurosurgeons or plastic surgeons.

I must add, that as with most scales developed based on limited cases, such as the study above, authors may tend to simplify or stratify patient characteristics into certain groups without any validation. Ideally, a scale or system should be developed and then tested to establish the utility of the scale in terms of generalizability and reproducibility in the hands of all potential users. I don't think the above system could be readily utilized by pediatricians, for example, in a meaningful way that could affect patient management. Furthermore, a CT scan is almost never needed to distinguish between syndromic, positional, and other types of plagiocephaly. Therefore, I believe the scale has little real-world use which helps me understand why during my training and while in practice, I have never used this scale.

Dr. Doug Courtemanche

This papers primary benefit is the discussion of terminology and the sorting of descriptive from etiologic terms in the various clinical types of frontal plagiocephaly.

The details of the complex skull base analysis allow a better understanding of the three-dimensional changes affecting the orbit and the lateral part of anterior cranial base in all types of plagiocephaly.

Although not specifically stated, a better understanding of the pathoanatomy should lead to a better plan for treatment.

The paper also provides a baseline for definition of abnormalities that can be followed post-treatment when objectively assessing results.

Protruding Ears—Pitfalls and Shortcomings

What It Classifies

Unfavorable results following otoplasty performed for outstanding or protruding ears.

System

Category A: Outline of ear is abnormal from the front view, with a major portion of the helix disappearing behind the reconstructed antihelix. A "disappearing helix."

Category B: Ear still protrudes or hangs out at top.

Category C: Ear still protrudes at top and bottom, and is overcorrected in the mid-portion. A "telephone ear."

Category D: Ear is overcorrected throughout, appearing somewhat "plastered" to the head.

Reference

McDowell AJ. Goals in otoplasty for protruding ears. *Plast Recon Surg.* 1968;41(1):17.

Uses

Primary: Description, Diagnosis, Etiology

Secondary: Research

Limited/none: Prognosis, Treatment

Comments

Dr. Paul Oxley

This classification, written in 1968, addresses what went wrong in a surgical correction. Very few classifications are designed to look at the outcome of an operation, generally choosing to look at the preoperative state and helping to plan treatment. This classification tries and succeeds in providing a framework to critically appraise the outcome of otoplasty for prominent ears.

It has limited use in research as it is a very subjective system. It would be improved by adding normal values to indicate overcorrection. Its main role is in describing the appearance following repair and the most obvious problem with the result. It clearly shows the location of the problem but does not in itself offer solutions to the problem. These solutions would depend largely on the original procedure and, more specifically, what was done to reshape the cartilage (eg, scoring techniques versus suture techniques).

Dr. Oscar M. Ramirez

Despite that this classification was described in an old article, it is still current in its applications. The different postoperative deformities outlined in categories A through D are still seen very frequently in our patients. This indicates that no significant progress has been made in this field. One important article that deals with one of the most frequent causes of this postoperative shortcomings is the one described by Bruce Bauer, David Song, and Margueritte Aitken in the article entitled "Combined Otoplasty Technique: Chondrocutaneous Conchal Resection as the Cornerstone for Correction of the Prominent Ear." *Plastic Reconstructive Surgery.* 110(4):1033-1040, September 2, 2002. I recommend its reading.

Prominent Ears

What It Classifies

Different forms of prominent ears.

System

See Table 3-6.

Reference

Graham KE and Gault DT. Endoscopic assisted otoplasty: a preliminary report. *Br J Plast Surg.* 1997;50:47.

Uses

Primary: Treatment, Description, Etiology

Secondary: Diagnosis, Research

Limited/none: Prognosis

Comments

Dr. Paul Oxley

This classification was developed to help the authors evaluate ears prior to apply-

Table 3–6. Prominent Ears

Type I	Deep concha with well developed antihelical fold. (a) No prominence of lobule (b) Prominent lobule not corrected by finger pressure
Type II	Poorly developed antihelix with or without deep concha. One crus poorly formed. (a) Finger pressure on helical rim corrects lobule prominence (b) Lobule prominence not corrected by finger pressure on rim
Type III	Absent antihelix fold between scaphal and conchal cartilages in the middle third of the ear. One or both crura absent. (a) Creation of antihelix by finger pressure on rim also corrects lobule (b) Lobule prominence not corrected by finger pressure
Type IV	Complex deformity (eg, lop ear)

ing endoscopic techniques. Although this is a very common condition, there are very few classifications that try to describe the problem. Most view the condition as one of either lack of the antihelical fold or prominence of the conchal bowl. Graham and Gault tried to better define the condition.

It is useful for stratification of patients prior to treatment and is fairly objective making it good for research and clinical applications. The system does not address the degree of deformity; it does try to stratify this based on the lobule. The specific treatment for a given problem is highly variable. Many techniques exist for each, all of which have shown both good and bad results.

Dr. Don Lalonde

Classifications are only valuable in my view if they serve to improve communication about treatment.

One good part of this prominauris classification is that it talks about digital pressure. One of the most significant recent advances in otoplasty surgery is that otoplasty is often not necessary if

babies with prominauris are splinted shortly after birth. The most important predicting factor in determining if splints will work is whether or not the deformity can be corrected with digital pressure. The same principle generally applies to prominauris surgery. If the deformity can be completely corrected with digital pressure, then sutures alone will likely do the trick. If digital pressure does not completely correct the deformity, then cartilage remodeling with cutting or scoring will often be required to make the ear look closer to normal.

I am not convinced that there is any value in separating types II and III of this classification. However, type I needs a conchal wedge resection, conchal scoring plus or minus sutures, or conchamastoid sutures. I prefer conchal wedge excision as conchamastoid sutures distort the external auditory meatus. Type II needs scaphal conchal sutures or scoring of the anterior of the antihelix, or a combination of the two. I prefer scaphal conchal sutures with no skin excision.

Lobule prominence can usually be corrected with either sutures or posterior skin excision or both. I prefer sutures.

Congenital Defects of Scalp and Calvarium

What It Classifies

Congenital scalp and calvarium bone deficiencies.

System

See Table 3-7.

Reference

Perlyn CA, Schmelzer R, Govier D, Marsh JL. Congenital scalp and calvarial deficiencies: principles for classification and surgical management. *Plast Reconstr Surg.* 2005; 115(4):1129-1141.

Uses

Primary: Diagnosis, Description, Research, Treatment

Secondary: Prognosis

Limited/none: Etiology

Comments

Dr. Paul Oxley

Congenital defects of the scalp or calvaria are rare and pose a significant challenge to the reconstructive surgeon. Significant morbidity can arise from this condition. Multiple techniques exist for both scalp and calvarial reconstruction and the choice depends largely on the extent of the problem and which tissues are missing.

Table 3-7. Scalp and Calvarium Defects

Class	Description
I	Open defects of the scalp alone
	A. Less than 2 cm in diameter
	B. Two to 5 cm in diameter
	C. Greater than 5 cm in diameter
II	Open defects of the skull alone
	A. Less than 2 cm in diameter
	B. Two to 5 cm in diameter
	C. Greater than 5 cm in diameter
	D. Any above size with:
	(+) herniated meningeal/ neural tissue
	(−) no herniated meningeal/neural tissue
III	Open defects of the skull and scalp
	A. Less than 2 cm in diameter
	B. Two to 5 cm in diameter
	C. Greater than 5 cm in diameter
	D. Any above size with:
	(+) herniated meningeal/ neural tissue
	(−) no herniated meningeal/neural tissue

This classification system is a descriptive classification based on defect type, location, size, and involvement of neurologic tissue. It was designed to help the surgeon develop a comprehensive care plan, both in the choice of reconstructive options and the timing of their implementation. The original article sets forth a treatment algorithm and is not covered in this review.

This is a very easy system to understand and use. It presents a clear picture of the defect in question and is clearly progressive. The higher the class, the more severe the defect. Prognosis is easily extrapolated from the classification. The exact etiology of the defects is not included this classification.

Tanzer Classification of Auricular Defects

What It Classifies

Congenital deformations and malformations of the ear.

System

Type I: Anotia

Type II: Complete hypoplasia (microtia)
   A Microtia with atresia of the external auditory meatus
   B Microtia without atresia of the external auditory meatus

Type III: Hypoplasia of the middle third of the auricle

Type IV: Hypoplasia of the superior third of the auricle
   A Constricted (cup or lop) ear
   B Cryptotia
   C Hypoplasia if the entire superior third of the auricle

Type V: Outstanding or prominent ear

Reference

Tanzer RC. Congenital deformities of the auricle. In: Converse JM, ed. *Reconstruc-tive Plastic Surgery.* 2nd ed. Philadelphia, Pa: WB Saunders; 1977: Chap. 35.

Uses

Primary: Diagnosis, Description, Research

Secondary: Treatment, Prognosis

Limited/none: Etiology

Comments

Dr. Paul Oxley

Over the years there have been many classification systems for auricular defects both prior to and since Tanzer developed his classification. Although some like Marx's (1926) are simpler and others are more complex (Weerda, 1988), Tanzer's seems to be the one that most people use.

This is a very comprehensive clinical classification of congenital auricular anomalies. It presents the varying conditions as a spectrum of conditions with most severe being the first type. In contrast, most classification systems assign a higher number to the more severe deformity.

The system lacks a little definition with respect to describing the severity of the condition and, as with outstanding ears, the anatomic cause of the deformity. Treatment varies by age and severity, and most have more than one option. The system does not go into etiology of the defect.

Dr. Gordon Wilkes

The true benefit of a classification system is to properly categorize a deformity, allow treatment planning, and carry out reconstruction. Now in the era of evidence-based medicine, the role of the classification system goes one step further. It should allow a basis for treatment outcomes to be measured and compared based on the original classification system. Then the classification system is most meaningful.

This is a classification system for congenital ear defects only. It is a system that differentiates into major ear deformities but does not further classify within each group. This classification system is helpful in the broadest terms for treatment planning. It is a classification for "lumpers rather than splitters!" The numbering within the Tanzer system although differentiating overall degree of severity, is not particularly helpful for classification or planning. The system is helpful in including constricted, lop, and cup ear. This is often a source of confusion for many.

Further classification systems have been developed within some of these numbered groupings by Dr. Tanzer and others, to more accurately differentiate among defects and be helpful for treatment planning. For example, Dr. Tanzer's classification of constricted ears is helpful to more carefully analyze and describe the defect and then plan appropriate reconstruction. Other classification systems have been developed for prominent ears, and microtia to correct for these shortcomings.

A more comprehensive classification system is needed that can categorize all types of major ear deformities regardless of etiology to allow comparison of treatment approaches and reconstructive results.

Tessier Classification of Craniofacial Clefts

What It Classifies

Facial clefts (not including cleft lip and palate).

AKA

Tessier Classification

System

The system divides facial and cranial clefts. Facial clefts (1–7) extend down from the orbit whereas cranial clefts (8–14) extend upward. A midline cleft is numbered 0. For facial clefts, as the number increases, the distance laterally from the midline increases, whereas for cranial clefts the opposite is true. When facial clefts extend into cranial clefts, the number usually adds up to 14. A 30 cleft is a midline cleft of the mandible. The cleft can affect any or all layers of the face. The soft tissue defect does not always correspond to bony cleft. This list is not comprehensive for all forms of rare facial clefts (Fig 3–9).

Cleft 0: Midline, aka median craniofacial dysraphia, goes through nasal bones, frontal bone, columella, lip, and maxilla. May be associated with hypertelorism or encephalocele (Fig 3–10).

Cleft 1: Between frontal process of maxilla and nasal bone and through the maxilla between the incisors. Aka paramedian craniofacial dysraphia, may be associated

with hypertelorism, widened nasal bridge, absent nasal bone, or bifid nasal dome.

Cleft 2: Cleft is lateral to cleft 1 at lateral incisor. Hypoplastic alar rim, hypertelorism, and wide, flat nasal bridge.

Cleft 3: Oculonasal cleft, running between the lateral incisor and canine into the maxilla and through the nasal and lacrimal bones. Medial wall of orbit and lacrimal apparatus may be deficient. Medial coloboma may be present.

Cleft 4: Runs from medial orbit to area between lateral incisor and canine without involving medial wall of maxilla (piriform aperture). Presence of lip cleft between philtral column and modeolus (meloschisis). Aka oculofacial 1 cleft.

Cleft 5: Most rare cleft. Runs lateral to inferior orbital foramen to corner of mouth. "Microeye" appearance. Central coloboma may be present. Aka oculofacial 2 cleft.

Cleft 6: Between maxilla and zygoma (which may be hypoplastic or absent). Associated with lateral lower lid colobomas and anti-mongoloid slant. When combined with clefts 7 and 8 forms part of Treacher-Collins syndrome. No soft tissue oral component.

Cleft 7: Most common facial cleft. Between zygoma, temporal bone, and behind maxillary alveolus.

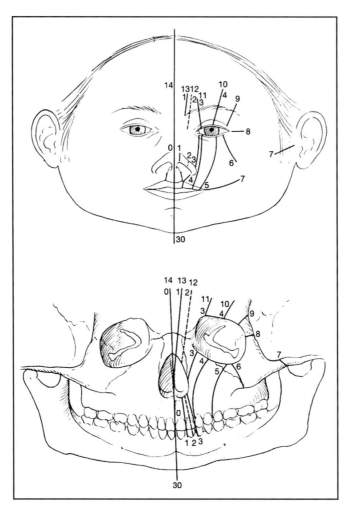

Fig 3–9. Tessier facial clefts. Tessier P. Anatomical classification of facial, craniofacial, and laterofacial clefts. *J Maxillofac Surg.* 1976;4:69. Copyright 1976 by Lippincott, Williams & Wilkins. Reprinted with permission.

May result in macrostomia. Also associated with microtia, mandibular dysplasia, canted occlusal plane, skin tags, and parotid gland abnormalities.

Cleft 8: Passes outward from lateral canthus. Extend between the zygoma and temporal bone in to the greater wing of the sphenoid. Rarely seen in isolation.

Cleft 9: Rarest cranial cleft. Extends from supraorbital position laterally. Associated with facial cleft 5.

Cleft 10: Extends from supraorbital position more medial than cleft 9. Associated with facial cleft 4.

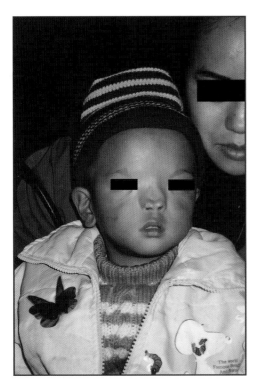

Fig 3–10. Tessier cleft 0.

May include encephalocele or hypertelorism.

Cleft 11: Extends from supra-orbital position more medial than cleft 10. Associated with facial cleft 3. May include encephalocele or hypertelorism.

Cleft 12: Created by agenesis of bone or abundance of cranial tissue. Does not involve orbit. Extension of facial cleft 2. May cause hypotelorism in the case of agenesis.

Cleft 13: Created by agenesis of bone or abundance of cranial tissue. Extension of facial cleft 1. May cause hypotelorism in the case of agenesis.

Cleft 14: Midline cleft. Created by agenesis of bone or abundance of cranial tissue. Extension of facial cleft 0. May cause either hyper-telorism or hypotelorism in the case of agenesis.

Cleft 30: Cleft of the mandible and lower lip. May be inferior extension of cleft 0. May in severe cases extend into neck and sternum.

References

Hobar PC. Craniofacial anomalies II: syndromes and surgery. *Selected Readings in Plastic Surgery.* 1994;7(25):1.

Tessier P. Anatomical classification of facial, craniofacial, and laterofacial clefts. *J Maxillofac Surg.* 1976;4:69.

Uses

Primary: Description, Research, Diagnosis

Secondary: Treatment, Prognosis

Limited/none: Etiology

Comments

Dr. Paul Oxley

Rare facial clefts are not the same as the more common cleft lip and palate, although they often coexist. It refers to congenital conditions effecting the soft tissue and bony structure of the face other than the more common cleft lip and palate. Although most are rarely seen, some well-known conditions, such as Treacher-Collins syndrome and macro-stomia are forms of facial clefts. When discussing facial clefts, there is a wide range of severity and the treatment in dependent on both this and the location of the cleft.

This classification is easily one of the most daunting and difficult to learn in plastic surgery. Nevertheless, once learned it is easy to apply and gives a clear diagnosis to other surgeons. Its biggest shortfall is that the soft tissue defect and the bony defect do not always coincide. In addition, several clefts may occur at the same time, as is the case with Treacher-Collins.

The key point is understanding that the facial and cranial components usually add up to 14. It is easiest to remember if one looks at which clefts affect the piriform aperture, mouth and orbit, and which teeth are involved in the case of the facial clefts.

Dr. Kevin L. Bush

This is an extremely useful classification originally defined by Tessier and based strictly on a clinical assessment of patients. The classification is useful for craniofacial clefts which may present with a spectrum of abnormality from severe to mild. The descriptive nature of the classification directs clinicians to specific abnormalities in bone, soft tissue, and other structures which may need to be addressed to treat these particular patients.

From a research point of view it has been useful in terms of grouping certain spectrums of individuals into descriptive groups. However, I feel it is only very useful for facial clefts and is not applicable to many other syndromes. This classification is the most useful when treating clinical patients and it is certainly the most commonly used classification for craniofacial clefts.

Van der Meulen's Craniofacial Dysplasia

What It Classifies

Dysplastic conditions including clefts of the facial skeleton using a focal fetal dysplasia model.

System

See Figure 3–11.

References

Hobar PC. Craniofacial anomalies II: syndromes and surgery. *Selected Readings in Plastic Surgery.* 1994;7(25):1.

van der Meulen JC, Mazzola R, Vermey-Keers C, et al. A morphogenetic classification of craniofacial malformations. *Plast Reconstr Surg.* 1983;71:560.

Uses

Primary: Etiology, Description, Diagnosis

Secondary: Research

Limited/none: Treatment, Prognosis

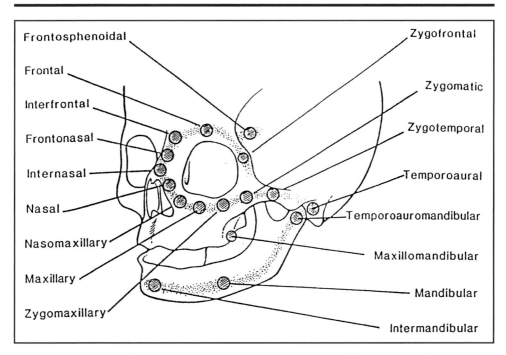

Fig 3–11. Craniofacial dysplasias. Hobar PC. Craniofacial anomalies II: syndromes and surgery. *Selected Readings in Plastic Surgery.* 1994;7(25):4. Copyright 1994 by Selected Readings in Plastic Surgery. Reprinted with permission.

Comments

Dr. Paul Oxley

This classification designed by van der Meulen and colleagues in 1983 looks at the cause of craniofacial clefts. The classification tries to correlate clinical features of a given condition with an embryogenic event. The classification uses the term "focal fetal dysplasia" as opposed to cleft when describing an arrest in the development of bone, skin, or muscle. Each anomaly is thus named after the area of arrest.

Van der Meulen and colleagues lay the craniofacial skeleton out as a helix (or "S" pattern on the left hemifacial skeleton). Along this course there are 17 points where they believe an arrest can happen. The system does allow for more than one area of arrest.

What separates this classification from the Tessier classification is that this system links an embryonic event to what is seen clinically. It helps the clinician to better understand the events leading up to the anomaly and how those events affect the facial skeleton. It does not attempt to further classify as to the cause of the embryonic event (chemical, genetic, etc). It does not help the clinician to determine treatment or predict prognosis as it does not describe the severity of the condition.

Dr. Kevin L. Bush

This classification is a relatively complicated classification that tries to delineate an event that occurs in embryologic development which could subsequently account for the abnormalities one sees in the pediatric and adult facial skeleton.

I personally have not found this classification particularly useful in the clinical situation.

Although this classification may be useful in further understanding the relationship of congenital abnormalities and to embryology, I have not found it useful either for determining treatment nor in the development of further research. Many craniofacial conditions do not have a single event clearly causing the developmental abnormalities seen.

Veau Classification

What It Classifies

Clefts of the secondary and primary palates starting posteriorly.

System

See Table 3-8.

References

Muzaffar AR, Byrd HS, Rohrich RJ, et al. Incidence of cleft palate fistula: an institutional experience with two-stage palatal repair. *Plast Reconstr Surg.* 2001;108(6): 1515-1518.

Veau V. *Division Palatine.* Paris: Masson: 1931.

Uses

Primary: Description, Diagnosis

Secondary: Research, Treatment

Limited/none: Etiology, Prognosis

Comments

Dr. Paul Oxley

Cleft lip and palate are some of the most common congenital problems seen by Plastic Surgeons. They vary from the simple to the complex and have had many surgeries created to correct them both. Classifying these clefts can be done in

Table 3-8. Veau Classification of Cleft Lip and Palate

Class	Site of Cleft
1	Soft palate
2	Soft and hard palate
3	Soft and hard palate and unilateral prepalatal cleft
4	Soft and hard palate and bilateral prepalatal clefts

Source: From "Incidence of cleft palate fistula: an institutional experience with two-stage palatal repair," Muzaffar AR, Byrd HS, Rohrich RJ, et al., *Plast Reconstr Surg.* 2001;108(6), pp.1515-1518. Copyright 2001 by Lippincott, Williams & Wilkins. Reprinted with permission.

many different ways. Most systems divide the primary palate (lip and palate anterior to incisive foramen) and secondary palate (remaining hard and soft palate) into two groups.

Veau's classification is one of the original attempts at defining clefts. Although most classifications start anteriorly, for example the Kernahan striped-Y, Veau views a cleft from the inside out, starting at the soft palate.

The classification system categorizes clefts of the secondary palate by treatment area and complexity. Type I is the easiest of the four to repair. The scheme is easy to learn and apply, and is universally understood. It does have significant limitations that limits use in research and planning treatment. It leaves out some information, such as the location of the cleft relative to the vomer, and does not include clefts of the primary palate. It also does not include overt or occult submucous clefts. In addition, some believe that the repair of cleft palate with respect to velophayngeal insufficiency switches the order of types II and III.

For the student learning about cleft lip and palate, this is a good system to start with to understand the basic types, but much greater knowledge will be expected with time.

Chapter 4

COSMETIC

Crow's Feet

What It Classifies

Pattern of crow's feet in the Caucasian female population.

System

1. Full fan pattern—crinkling of the lateral canthal skin from lower lateral brow, across the upper eyelid, past lateral canthus, and across the lower lid /cheek junction.
2. Lower lid/cheek area alone
3. Limited to upper eyelid skin down to lateral canthus
4. Limited to area around lateral canthus

Reference

Kane MAC. Classification of crow's feet patterns among Caucasian women: the key to individualizing treatment. *Plast Reconstr Surg*. 2003(suppl);112(5):33S–39S.

Uses

Primary: Diagnosis, Research

Secondary: Prognosis, Description

Limited/none: Etiology, Treatment

Comments

Dr. Paul Oxley

Crow's feet are a common cause of cosmetic concern. Typically used as a term to identify wrinkles radiating from the lateral canthus, these wrinkles often occur in tandem with other periorbital wrinkles. Many treatments have been proposed to correct these wrinkles; however, like most areas in cosmetic surgery, the treatments have variable success. It is important to differentiate the cause and extent of a problem before applying a treatment method. It is also important to have standard definitions for a condition to properly compare results.

This paper sets forth a classification of the patterns of animation and the subsequent crow's feet. The findings are that the patterns described happened in decreasing frequency and require different therapeutic strategies. Asymmetric patterns were found in roughly 6% of people, and age was not a contributing factor.

This classification is useful for diagnosing the pattern of wrinkles around the lateral canthus. However, as it is based on the Caucasian female population it has limited application. It does not describe the severity or extent of the wrinkles so by itself has difficulty describing the wrinkles in any given patient. It is a useful start to research into effective therapeutic options for this area, but does not by itself help to direct treatment.

Face Lift (Baker)

What It Classifies

Patient types for short scar facelifts.

System

See Table 4–1.

References

Baker DC. Minimal incision rhytidectomy (short scar face lift) with lateral SMASec-tomy: evolution and application. *Aesthetic Surg J.* 2001;21:14

Gryskiewicz JM. Submental suction assisted lipectomy without platysmaplasty: pushing the (skin) envelope to avoid a face lift for unsuitable candidates. *Plast Reconstr Surg.* 2003;112(5):1393–1405.

Uses

Primary: Description, Diagnosis

Secondary: Research, Treatment

Limited/none: Prognosis, Etiology

Table 4–1. Baker Face Lift Score

	Baker Type			
	I	II	III	IV
Age	40s	late 40–50	late 50–60	60s to 70s
Jowls	Early	Moderate	Significant	Significant
Submental Fat	±	+	+	+
Laxity	Slight	Moderate	Moderate	Deep creases
Elasticity	Good	Poor	Poor	Poor

Comments

Dr. Paul Oxley

Baker's assessment tool for short scar facelifts can be applied to either the short or long scar techniques. It is a clear and concise system for evaluating patients prior to facelift.

Its weaknesses are based largely on the fact that so many variables exist. For example, age does not necessarily correlate with any of the other characteristics. This leaves the problem of defining the individual who spans more than one group. It is a useful tool for directing treatment. As a research tool it is limited for the reasons mentioned above, but can still convey adequate information about patients entered into a study and their responses to treatment.

Dr. Don Guichon

This classification reflects Dr. Baker's style. It is straightforward, intuitive, and useful. It is safe, readily understood, and a "take home" that can be put into effect immediately. Dr Baker's practical approach to facial aging is easy to apply and to relate to any surgeon's personal preferences of surgery. It probably is not comprehensive enough for the researcher to compare subtle nuances of technique. However, for the everyday plastic surgeon it is very workable. It can be applied to primary and secondary facelifts.

Facial Wrinkling (Fitzpatrick)

What It Classifies

Perioral and periorbital wrinkling and skin aging.

System

I Fine wrinkles, mild elastosis
  ■ Fine textural changes with subtly accentuated skin lines

II Fine to moderate wrinkles, moderate number of lines, moderate elastosis
  ■ Distinct papular elastosis, individual papules with yellow translucency, dyschromia

III Fine to deep wrinkles, numerous lines ± redundant skin, severe elastosis
  ■ Multipapular and confluent elastosis, thickened yellow and pallid cutis rhomboidalis

References

Fitzpatrick's classification of facial wrinkling (perioral and periorbital). From: Lemperle G., Holmes RE, Cohen SR, Lemperle SM, A classification of facial wrinkles, *Plast Reconstr Surg.* 2001;108(6):1735–1750.

Fitzpatrick RE, Goldman MP, Satur NM, Tope WD. Pulsed carbon dioxide laser resurfacing of photo-aged facial skin. *Arch Dermatol.* 1996;132:395.

Uses

Primary: Description, Diagnosis

Secondary: Treatment

Limited/none: Research, Etiology, Prognosis

Comments

Dr. Paul Oxley

The treatment of wrinkles is one of the central parts of an aesthetic surgeon's reason for being. As one of the most common reasons why people seek facial rejuvenation there have been many treatments developed over the years for wrinkles. The question is how best to treat them.

Like most problems in surgery, once the cause of the problem is known, the treatment is easier to determine. Fitzpatrick attempts to categorize different degrees of wrinkles and correlate them to other findings in the surrounding skin. By focusing on the periorbital and perioral regions, he is looking at a very difficult area to treat and maintain long-lasting effect. This system includes the microscopic changes associated with different degrees of wrinkling. Although allowing a physician or surgeon to understand the underlying histology of the wrinkles it does not have immediate clinical application. It has not been directly linked to treatment methods and long-term outcome studies.

Dr. Don Guichon

This is a nice attempt to correlate clinical observation to underlying dermal pathology. This is, however, probably overly simplified, as really its only application is to resurfacing modalities. It is not applicable to the full range of the armamentarium of the plastic surgeon to correct the concerns of the aging process. That said, it does create a simple and useful numeric method of evaluating results of ablative procedures.

Facial Wrinkling (Lemperle)

What It Classifies

The degree of severity of facial wrinkles.

System

Location of wrinkle:

- Horizontal forehead lines
- Glabellar frown lines
- Periorbital lines
- Preauricular lines
- Cheek lines
- Nasolabial folds
- Radial upper lip lines
- Radial lower lip lines
- Corner of the mouth lines
- Marionette lines
- Labiomental crease
- Horizontal neck folds

See Table 4-2.

Reference

Lemperle G, Holmes RE, Cohen SR, Lemperle SM. A classification of facial wrinkles. *Plast Reconstr Surg.* 2001;108(6):1735-1750.

Uses

Primary: Description, Diagnosis, Research

Secondary:

Limited/none: Treatment, Etiology, Prognosis

Table 4–2. Facial Wrinkles (Lemperle)

Class	Description
0	No wrinkles
1	Just perceptible wrinkle
2	Shallow wrinkle
3	Moderately deep wrinkle
4	Deep wrinkle, well-defined edges
5	Very deep wrinkle, redundant fold

Source: From "A classification of facial wrinkles," by Lemperle G, Holmes RE, Cohen SR, Lemperle SM. *Plast Reconstr Surg.* 2001;108(6): 1735–1750. Copyright 2001 by Lippincott, Williams & Wilkins. Reprinted with permission.

Comments

Dr. Paul Oxley

Facial wrinkling is a concern to many aesthetic surgeons and dermatologists. The challenge is to determine which treatment is best for any given patient. To reach a decision, the surgeon must know what works best for different degrees of facial wrinkling. There have been other attempts to classify facial wrinkling, including Fitzpatrick and Hamilton. The Fitzpatrick system focuses on the appearance of both the wrinkle itself and the skin changes associated with it. Hamilton's system addresses the cause of facial wrinkles or folds and suggests treatments.

Lemperle's classification attempts to classify the severity of the wrinkle without identifying the cause or effect. It does not suggest specific treatments for the different levels or classes. What it does provide is a useful tool for diagnosis and description, by categorizing each of the anatomic areas commonly affected by wrinkling and grading the wrinkles at each. This allows for easy interpretation, and it is very reliable and reproducible in the case of research. This tool can be used in longitudinal studies, multicenter comparisons, or individual clinical assessment. It is easily used by anyone from a medical student to an experienced dermatologist, or surgeon.

Dr. Don Guichon

This classification is a nice attempt to take what we see and quantitate it. As such it is a valid attempt to take an observed, artistic impression and create a numeric scale. It is not probably something that one would use from day to day. However, if one were to link it to treatment modalities, or personal preferences of treatment, it would become a useful documentary tool. It could become a nice reference for charting if the locations were transposed to a picture (eg, using Fig. 2 in Lemperle's original article).

Fitzpatrick Classification

What It Classifies

The skin's photoaging tendency with respect to skin pigmentation and inherent ability to tan.

System

See Table 4–3.

References

Barton Jr FE. The aging face: rejuvenation surgery and adjunctive measures. *Selected Readings in Plastic Surgery*. 1997;8(19):1.

Fitzpatrick TB. The validity and practicality of sun-reactive skin types I through VI. *Arch Dermatol*. 1988;124:869

Table 4–3. Fitzpatrick Photoaging Scale

Type	Color	Reaction to 1st Summer Exposure
I	White	Always burns and never tans
II	White	Usually burns, tans with difficulty
III	White	Sometimes mild burn, tans average
IV	Moderate brown	Rarely burns, tans with ease
V	Dark brown	Very rarely burn, tans very easily
VI	Black	Never burns, tans very easily

Source: From "The aging face: rejuvenation surgery and adjunctive measures," Barton Jr FE, *Selected Readings in Plastic Surgery*. 1997;8(19). Copyright 1997 by Selected Readings in Plastic Surgery. Reprinted with permission.

Uses

Primary: Description

Secondary: Etiology, Treatment

Limited/none: Diagnosis, Research, Prognosis

Comments

Dr. Paul Oxley

Fitzpatrick's classification is one of the most commonly used in Aesthetic Der-matology and the treatment of skin cancer. It is used to describe skin types, and is easily applied by the clinician. Unfortunately, it is a subjective classification as it partly relies on the history given by the patient. For this reason it has a limited use in research.

Its main role in aesthetic surgery is in helping the clinician determine the appropriate chemical peel or laser treatment for a patient and the intensity and duration of that treatment. The absence of tanning ability correlates closely with a patient's sensitivity to chemical peels and dermabrasion.

Goglau Classification

What It Classifies

Actinic damage to the skin.

AKA

Goglau's Classification of Photoaging Groups

System

Type I: "No Wrinkles"
- Early photoaging
- Mild pigment changes
- No keratoses
- Minimal wrinkles
- Younger patient, 20s or 30s
- Minimal or no make-up
- No scarring (1990 paper)

Type II: "Wrinkles in Motion"
- Early to moderate photoaging
- Early senile lentigines visible
- Keratoses palpable but not visible
- Parallel smile lines beginning to appear
- Late 30s or 40s
- Usually wear some foundation
- Mild scarring (1990)

Type III: "Wrinkles at Rest"
- Advanced photoaging
- Obvious dyschromia, telangectasias
- Visible keratoses
- Wrinkles even when not moving
- Fifties or older
- Always wears heavy foundation
- Moderate acne scarring (1990)

Type IV: "Only Wrinkles"
- Severe photoaging
- Yellow-gray color of skin
- Actinic keratoses and skin cancer have occurred

- Wrinkling throughout, no normal skin
- Sixth or seventh decade
- Can't wear makeup, "cakes and cracks"
- Severe acne scarring (1990)

References

Barton Jr FE. The aging face: rejuvenation surgery and adjunctive measures. *Selected Readings in Plastic Surgery.* 1997;8(19):1.

Goglau RG. Presented at the Chemical Peel Symposium, American Academy of Dermatology, Atlanta, December 4, 1990.

Goglau RG. Chemical peeling and aging skin. *J Geri Dermatol.* 1994;2:30-35.

Uses

Primary: Description, Diagnosis

Secondary: Treatment, Research, Prognosis

Limited/none: Etiology

Comments

Dr. Paul Oxley

Goglau's classification system is used widely to help select options for facial rejuvenation. It has been modified slightly from its original version, excluding acne scarring. It looks at the degree of imperfection in the facial skin, and what steps are being taken to hide those by the patient. It helps to direct the choice for cosmetic rejuvenation from peels and injectables to lasers or surgery. Its biggest challenge lies in its application to those patients who may cross over between groups. As the classification deals with photoaging changes to skin, etiology is the same for each group.

Dr. Paul L. Schnur

The Goglau classification of actinic damage to the face is straightforward. However, it has enough elements to make it difficult to remember. In my experience most clinicians judge the degree of severity without the use of a classification system. In my practice I record severity of actinic damage by a description of the findings recorded in my clinical notes. If necessary I supplement the notes by photographs. I have not observed many plastic surgeons use this classification in their clinical practice. It is quite possible that dermatologists find this classification helpful in their daily care of patients.

If one is planning a research project on patients with actinic changes of the face this might be a worthwhile classification so that patients can be grouped into levels of severity.

As far as the clinical care of the patient is concerned I feel that a careful description of the patients findings supplemented by quality photographs it the most accurate method of describing the severity of the problem.

Male Pattern Baldness

What It Classifies

Male pattern baldness using letters form the English language as analogous shapes. It also describes anterior hairline shape as a separate classification tied to the first.

System

Basic Shapes: M, C, O, U, MO, CO

Anterior hairline shape:

A. Linear

B. Linear with central protrusion

C. Round

D. Round with central protrusion.

Reference

Note. Portions of this section were taken from "A new classification of male pattern baldness and a clinical study of the anterior hairline," Koo S-H, Chung H-S, Yoon E-S, Park S-H, *Aesth Plast Surg.* 2000;24, pp. 46–51. Copyright 2000 by Springer Science and Business Media. Reprinted with kind permission of Springer Science and Business Media.

Uses

Primary: Description, Diagnosis

Secondary: Treatment, Research

Limited/none: Prognosis, Etiology

Comments

Dr. Paul Oxley

Male pattern baldness is one of the most common reasons for men to seek out aesthetic procedures. The presence and appearance of scalp hair is a key component in making a man look and feel young. Although gray hair is easily colored, baldness is much more difficult to treat. Whereas wigs and comb-overs have been the treatment of choice in the past, surgical techniques have become more common in recent decades. These have evolved from strip grafts and plugs to the micrografts used today.

It is easy to document that a patient is bald but it is much more difficult to accurately reflect the pattern of hair loss on paper. Norwood was the first to develop a widely accepted method of describing the pattern of male baldness. His system, also described in this book is very comprehensive though difficult to remember by the casual user. Koo et al attempted to define baldness using a simplified system that uses letters of the alphabet whose shape matches that of the balding hair line. It is easy to imagine how the receding hairline can be compared to one of the letters above, with the "O" representing the bald patch with an intact anterior hairline. This is where the shape of the anterior line also needs to be recorded. For the casual user, this system is more easily remembered. It does not have the exactness of Norwood's classification but is easily reproduced.

It does not delve into the cause, though in male pattern baldness this information is rarely of significance in determining prognosis or treatment. This system also does not describe the severity of the problem, something done by the Norwood classification.

Norwood Classification

What It Classifies

Most common types of male pattern baldness.

System

See Figure 4-1 and Figure 4-2.

References

Hubbard TJ. Hair restoration surgery. In: Georgiade GS, Riefkohl R & Levin LS, eds. *Georgiade Plastic, Maxillofacial and Reconstructive Surgery.* 3rd ed. Baltimore Md: Williams & Wilkins; 1997:667.

Norwood OT. Male pattern baldness: classification and incidence. *South Med J.* 1975; 68:1359.

Norwood OT, Shiell RC. *Hair Transplant Surgery.* 2nd ed. Springfield, Ill: Charles C. Thomas; 1984.

Unger WP. Treatment for Baldness. In: Aston SJ, Beasley RW, Thorne CHM, eds. *Grabb and Smith's Plastic Surgery.* 5th ed. Philadelphia, Pa: Lippincott-Raven Publishers; 1997:570.

Uses

Primary: Description, Diagnosis, Research

Secondary: Treatment, Prognosis

Limited/none: Etiology

Comments

Dr. Paul Oxley

The treatment of male pattern baldness is a huge industry in North America. Each year, millions of men try comb-overs and wigs to hide this problem. Many also turn to medications or surgery in an attempt to regain their hair. The treatment surgically depends, in part, on the extent and pattern of the baldness.

The Norwood classification was one of the first systems for grading and describing hair loss patterns. This classification is used extensively to help predict hair loss and possible treatment options.

The classification is picture based with an obvious progression through the system from mild to severe. Unfortunately, the pictures are hard to memorize for some, and unless a physician is using this system regularly, frequent referral to a chart is necessary. It has a high subjective component as the cutoff from one to the next is ill defined, so its ability to be used as a research tool is slightly limited.

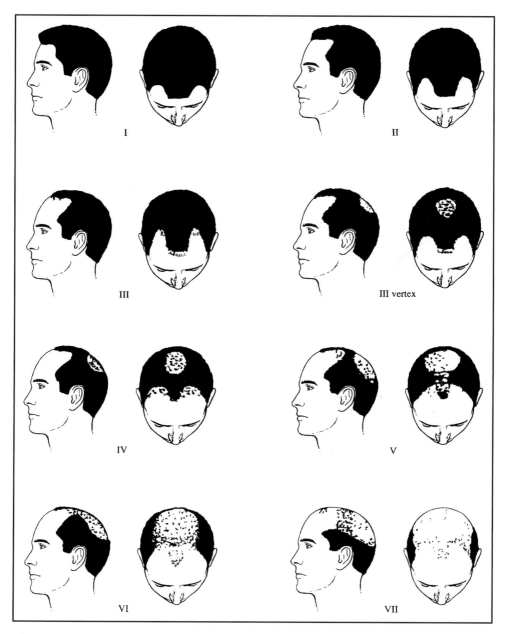

Fig 4–1. Norwood classification of male pattern baldness. Unger WP. Treatment for baldness. In: Aston SJ, Beasley RW, and Thorne CHM eds, *Grabb and Smith's Plastic Surgery,* 5th ed, Philadelphia, Pa: Lippincott Raven Publishers, 1997:570. Copyright 1997 by Lippincott, Williams & Wilkins. Reprinted with permission.

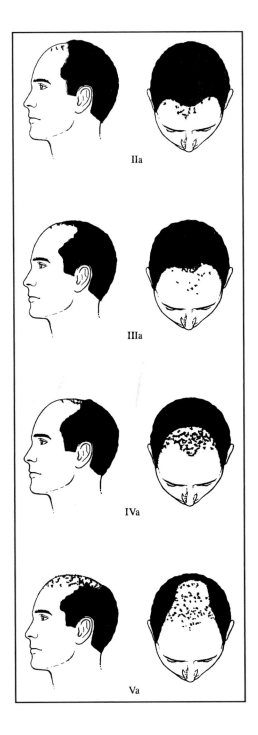

IIa

IIIa

IVa

Va

Fig 4–2. Norwood classification of male pattern baldness. Unger WP. Treatment for baldness. In: Aston SJ, Beasley RW, and Thorne CHM eds, *Grabb and Smith's Plastic Surgery*, 5th ed, Philadelphia Pa: Lippincott Raven Publishers, 1997:570. Copyright 1997 by Lippincott, Williams & Wilkins. Reprinted with permission.

Hamilton Classification

What It Classifies

Facial contour changes and their causes.

System

See Table 4–4.

References

Lemperle G, Holmes RE, Cohen SR, Lemperle SM. A classification of facial wrinkles. *Plast Reconstr Surg.* 2001;108(6):1735-1750.

Hamilton D. A classification of the aging face and its relationship to remedies. *J Cli. Dermatol.* 1998, Summer;35.

Uses

Primary: Description

Secondary: Research, Treatment, Diagnosis

Limited/none: Etiology, Prognosis

Comments

Dr. Paul Oxley

Facial aging is a common reason people have for seeing aesthetic surgeons. There are numerous treatments to correct the signs of aging; however, it can be difficult to determine which approach is best. The basic categories are those that work on the surface (laser, chemical peels), low invasive procedures such as Botox® and other injectables, and more invasive procedures such as facelifts and blepharoplasty. To achieve the best outcome for a patient the surgeon must select procedures that target the tissue responsible for the aging.

Table 4–4. Hamilton Classification

Facial Aging	Clinical Morphology	Tissue Location	Clinical Location	Optimal Etiology	Treatment
A	Folds	Muscular	Nasolabial folds, neck, eyelids	Loss of tone, gravity	Rhytidectomy blepharoplasty
B	Furrows	Musculo-cutaneous	Forehead, Smile lines	Repeated facial expressions	Fillers, injectables, implants
C	Wrinkles	Cutaneous	Cheeks, crows feet, perioral	Intrinsic aging, photoaging	Resurfacing laser, chemical peel
D	Combination				Combined approach

Source: From Hamilton D. A classification of the aging face and its relationship to remedies. *J Clin Dermatol.* 1998, Summer; p.35.

Hamilton describes the changes seen in the aging face and places them alongside the suspected cause of the problem. He divides these in to those caused by inherent skin changes, musculocutaneous changes, muscle changes, or a combination of the above. Hamilton also offers a basic selection of procedures to correct the appearance. In so doing he allows the surgeon to determine the cause specific to the problem and then determine the best treatment option.

The system is limited in that it only suggests the types of intervention that the surgeon should consider; this leaves many options from which to choose. It also leaves open the interpretation of a furrow versus a wrinkle versus a fold. In addition, it ignores severity as a key indicator of when to intervene. For example, the nasolabial fold is a normal anatomic structure that in some people becomes aesthetically concerning. When does it cross that line?

In all, this system is useful for categorizing the aging process and allowing readers and users to better understand the causes of facial aging.

Dr. Don Guichon

This is a simple, intuitive framework from which to work. It attempts to correlate the clinical morphology, the pathophysiology, and the treatment modalities. This is a classification for "lumpers." It is meant to be used as first approach to the problems of the aging face. As such it is a very good starting point for the beginner. As one gains experience, nuances will be gained that can be added to this framework. Personalization of this classification will make it a reliable part of the surgeon's practice.

Dermal Fillers

What It Classifies

U.S. FDA-approved injectables.

System

See Table 4-5.

Reference

Lemperle G, Rullan PP, Gauthier-Hazan N. Avoiding and treating dermal filler complications. *Plast Reconstr Surg.* 2006(Sept 1 suppl);118(3S):92S–107S.

Uses

Primary: Description

Secondary: Treatment, Research

Limited/none: Prognosis, Etiology, Diagnosis

Comments

Dr. Paul Oxley

This classification is based on the dermal fillers currently approved by the U.S. Food and Drug Administration and is not applicable to all countries. Knowledge of the available fillers in your area of practice is essential. This classification does provide a framework upon which to place those fillers available or approved in your area. This allows for easier understanding of the options available for any given problem and their likelihood of success.

Table 4–5. Dermal Fillers

Brand Name	Active Ingredient	Mechanism of Action	Bio-degradable	Persistence
Zyderm	Collagen	Volumizer	Yes	4 mo
Restylane	Hyaluronic acid	Volumizer	Yes	6 mo
ArteFill	PMMA	Stimulator	No	Permanent
Silikon 1000	Silicone	Volumizer	No	Permanent
Radiesse	Calcium Apatite	Volumizer	Yes	1 yr
Sculptra	PLLA	Stimulator	Yes	1 yr
Autol. Fat	Living Fat	Volumizer	Yes/no	Unpredictable

PMMA: polmethylmethacrylate; PLLA: poly-L-lactic acid.

At time of acceptance for publication in PRS, ArteFill's approval was pending.

Classification of U.S. Food and Drug Administration–Approved Injectables

Source: From "Avoiding and treating dermal filler complications," Lemperle G, Rullan PP, Gauthier-Hazan N, *Plast Reconstr Surg.* 2006;118(3S):92–107. Copyright 2006 by Lippincott, Williams & Wilkins. Reprinted with permission.

Dr. Nick Carr

This is an American perspective which, as a result, misses a few available elsewhere (eg, Bioalkamyd, Juvederm, Artecol).

This classification is not terribly useful in that there are many other parameters necessary in choosing the appropriate filler, including depth of injection, viscosity, and need for allergy testing. For the student studying for exams it gives a basic layout which may be useful but this is a rapidly changing field and will be constantly outdated.

Foreign Body Reactions

What It Classifies

Foreign body reaction by the body to implanted or injected materials.

System

See Table 4-6.

Table 4-6. Foreign Body Reaction

Grade	Pattern
I	Slight reaction with a few inflammatory cells
II	Clear inflammatory reaction with one or two giant cells
III	Fibrous tissue with inflammatory cells, lymphocytes, and giant cells
IV	Granuloma with encapsulated implants and clear foreign body reaction

Source: From "Human histology and persistence of various injectable filler substances for soft tissue augmentation," Lemperle G, Morhenn V, Charrier U. *Aesthetic Plastic Surgery.* 2003; 27(5):354–366. Copyright 2003 by Springer Science Business and Media. Reprinted with kind permission from Springer Science and Business Media.

References

Duranti F, Salti G, Bovani B, Calandra M, Rosati M. Injectable hyaluronic acid gel for soft tissue augmentation. *Dermatol Surg.* 1988;24:1317.

Lemperle G, Morhenn V, Charrier U. Human histology and persistence of various injectable filler substances for soft tissue augmentation. *Aesth Plast Surg.* 2003;27(5): 354-366.

Uses

Primary: Research, Description

Secondary: Diagnosis

Limited/none: Prognosis, Treatment, Etiology

Comments

Dr. Richard Crawford and Dr. Paul Oxley

Any substance placed in the body as a filler or implant will elicit a host response. The ideal substance would not generate any response unless desired to do so. There are no ideal substances. Currently approved fillers and implants have been developed and tested to ensure a negligible, or at least controlled, host response which results in an optimal clinical outcome. The host response to an injectable or implanted material can greatly affect the outcome of the treatment; idiosyncratic host responses can be difficult to predict. When doing any research on these substances, a common terminology is important to be able to compare research outcomes and treatment efficacy.

This classification looks at the histologic changes and host response to foreign bodies. It can be easily applied in any circumstance where tissue samples can be obtained. Grade I or II reactions are nonspecific and commonly occur not only in foreign-body reactions but also during repair reactions to surgery or other physical injuries, ischemia, infection, or endogenous inflammatory processes. In contrast, Grade III or IV reactions are relatively specific to either foreign-body reactions or infections, but sometimes the difference between foreign-body reaction and infection is difficult to determine on a histologic basis alone. If an infection is suspected, the histologic specimen should undergo special staining for organisms and fresh tissue should be submitted for bacterial, mycobacterial, and fungal culture.

The clinical significance of any given grade of reaction is not clear and will vary from patient to patient; for this reason this classification is not routinely used by surgical pathologists when reporting on tissue removed during the clinical care of patients.

Injectable Fillers

What It Classifies

Different types of injectable substances based on their histologic reaction pattern.

System

1. Autologous fat rarely is permanent and its fate is unpredictable. The mechanism for long-term survival of fat or stem cells has yet to be understood.
2. Natural filler substances such as collagen and hyaluronic acids are phagocytosed slowly with minimal histologic reaction.
3. Fluid filler substances, such as fluid silicone and acrylamides, cause little fibrosis but can dislocate larger volumes through muscle movement and gravity; they are considered dead implants.
4. Particulate materials like PMA gravel and PLA microspheres are packed and induce minimal foreign-body reaction and fibrosis. They are pure fillers and are slowly resorbed.
5. Microspheres from nonresorbable PMMA or resorbable dextran are stimulants for encapsulation and scaffolds of permanent or temporary connective tissue formation, considered living implants.

References

Duranti F, Salti G, Bovani B, Calandra M, Rosati M. Injectable hyaluronic acid gel for soft tissue augmentation. *Dermatol Surg.* 1998;24:1317.

Lemperle G, Morhenn V, Charrier U. Human histology and persistence of various injectable filler substances for soft tissue augmentation. *Aesth Plast Surg.* 2003;27(5): 354-366.

Uses

Primary: Research, Description, Prognosis, Treatment

Secondary:

Limited/none: Diagnosis, Etiology

Comments

Dr. Paul Oxley

Injectable materials cause a host response that ranges from mild to severe. It is important to understand the likely reactions to a substance to determine the likely outcome after treatment.

This classification addresses the early host response to different types of injectables. It was created by looking at histologic samples of various injectable materials and grouping the results. It considered biologic, artificial, permanent and resorbable materials. The host response varied by group and thus forms the classification.

This system is useful for grouping fillers and allowing results from one type to be compared to results from others or within a group. This is important in showing the superiority of one material over another for a given clinical problem. It is also useful in that it allows prediction of long-term results. Unfortunately, some late complications, such as granuloma formation are unpredictable and limit the usefulness of this classification.

Lateral Canthoplasty

What It Classifies

Different types of lateral canthoplasty for lower eyelid correction.

System

See Table 4-7.

Reference

Glat PM, Jelks GW, Jelks EB, Wood M, Gadangi P, Longaker MT. Evolution of the lateral canthoplasty: techniques and indications. *Plast Reconstr Surg.* 1997;100(6):1396-1405.

Uses

Primary: Description, Treatment

Secondary: Research

Limited/none: Prognosis, Etiology, Diagnosis

Comments

Dr. Paul Oxley

In this system the authors have looked at the ways to correct the position of the lower eyelid and have compiled a classification of the different procedures commonly used. Although assuming familiarity with each of the techniques mentioned, this system clearly lays out the options for a surgeon faced with a given clinical condition. It is a very useful system as well for those learning about lower eyelid correction as it helps teach an approach to the issue.

Table 4–7. Types of Lateral Canthoplasty

Procedure Code	Name of Procedure
1	Horizontal lid shortening with medial canthoplasty
2	Horizontal lid shortening with lateral canthal suspension
3	Complex lateral canthoplasty (for paralysis, anophthalmos, craniofacial
4	Lateral canthoplasty for prosthetic eye
5	Dermal orbicular pennant lateral canthoplasty
6	Inferior retinacular lateral canthoplasty
7A	Lateral canthoplasty with correction of retraction without skin graft
7B	Lateral canthoplasty with correction of retraction with skin graft

Source: From "Evolution of the lateral canthoplasty: techniques and indications," Glat PM, Jelks GW, Jelks EB, Wood M, Gadangi P, Longaker MT. *Plast Reconstr Surg.* 1997;100(6):1396–1405. Copyright 1997 by Lippincott, Williams & Wilkins. Reprinted with permission.

Male Foreheadplasty

What It Classifies

Different types of incisions in forehead rejuvenation in males.

System

See Table 4–8.

Reference

Connell BF, Marten TJ. The male forehead-plasty—recognizing and treating aging in the upper face. *Clin Plast Surg.* 1991; 18(4):653.

Uses

Primary: Description, Treatment

Secondary: Diagnosis

Limited/none: Etiology, Prognosis, Research

Comments

Dr. Paul Oxley

The choice of incision in open forehead rejuvenation or brow lift in male patients depends largely on the position of the anterior hairline and the presence and

Table 4–8. Male Forheadplasty Incisions

Type A:	Forehead (pretrichial) – follows natural undulations of the frontal hairline and then moves back into the temple hair to the root of the ear.
Type B:	Corobregmatic (coronal) – gull-wing-shaped posttrichial incision overlying coronal suture.
Type C:	Vertex – similar to corobregmatic but more posterior
Type D:	Lambdoidal – posteriorly placed coronal incision approximately two-thirds of the way between the forehead and the crown.
Type E:	W-incisions – for patients with balding at sides but low anterior hairline.
Type F:	Lambdoidal paddle – similar to Type B or C but allows for removal or reduction of occipital bald patch.
Type G:	Interlocking M's – V to Y advancements at apices of bald temporal scalp.

Source: From "The male foreheadplasty—recognizing and treating aging in the upper face," Connell BF, Marten TJ. *Clinics in Plastic Surgery.* 1991;18(4):653. Copyright 1991 by Elsevier. Reprinted with permission.

extent of baldness. This system includes the hair pattern and describes the different techniques used in brow lifts relative to those hair patterns. With the evolution and greater acceptance of the endoscopic forehead or brow lift, this classification has lost some of its use. Nevertheless, in the case of significant ptosis of the brow or deep forehead folds, the open technique can give remarkable results.

It is important to recognize the impact of baldness in these patients and to reduce that when possible, and to hide the scars in the most effective way.

This classification gives a framework for determining the best incisions and therefore directs treatment. It does nothing to convey a diagnosis and has no practical application in research.

Dr. Oscar M. Ramirez

This article is an excellent review and has become a landmark paper on male forehead rejuvenation. The classification system is helpful for planning and possibly of evaluation of the incisions used for foreheadplasty. The different types of incisions can be adapted to the different hairline types including those without a discernible clear hairline. However, with the advent and acceptance of the endoscopic forehead rejuvenation, many of the indications of this classification might need to be revised. Patients with male pattern baldness can be operated on using 1.5 to 2-cm slip incisions that when properly closed become invisible.

Midfacial Aging

What It Classifies

The degree of tissue ptosis in the midface and which surgery is indicated in addition to lower lid blepharoplasty.

System

See Table 4-9.

References

Hester TR, Codner MA, McCord CD. The "centrofacial" approach for correction of facial aging using the transblepharolplasty subperiosteal cheek lift. *Aesth Surg Quart.* 1996 Spring;16(1):81.

Flowers RS, Periorbital aesthetic surgery for men. Eyelids and related structures. *Clin Plast Surg.* 1991:18(4):689-729.

Uses

Primary: Diagnosis, Treatment

Secondary: Description

Limited/none: Etiology, Research, Prognosis

Comments

Dr. Paul Oxley

Hester, Codner, and McCord divide their patients based on this classification for

Table 4–9. Midfacial Aging

Class	Aging	Procedure
I	Confined to lower lid	Surgery confined to the lower lid; cheek lift not necessary
II	Early ptosis of the lid skin and malar soft tissue; nasolabial fold minimally affected	Indicated lower lid surgery plus cheek lift without rhytidectomy
III	Generalized facial aging	Indicated lower lid surgery plus cheek lift plus indicated rhytidectomy

Source: From "The 'centrofacial' approach for correction of facial aging using the transblepharolplasty subperiosteal cheek lift," Hester TR, Codner MA, McCord CD. *Aesthetic Surgery Quarterly.* 1996;16(1), p.81. Copyright 1996 by Elsevier. Reprinted with permission.

diagnostic and treatment planning purposes. It is devised to help determine the extent of the procedure required for a given aesthetic challenge. The paper describes each class more precisely in the text than it does in this table:

Class I: Lower eyelid changes with excess skin, muscle, or prominent orbital fat pads without significant ptosis of cheek skin, or infraorbital hollowness.

Class II: Limited ptosis of cheek skin and malar fat pad with thinning of the skin over the infraorbital rim; conspicuous tear trough with minimal or no exaggeration of the nasolabial fold (Flowers).

Class III: Generalized facial aging with more extensive ptosis of malar soft tissue with infraorbital hollowness and prominence of nasolabial fold. In addition, festoons or malar bags may be present.

The classification helps surgeons decide what procedure may be indicated but it leaves the type of operation up to the surgeon. It is a fairly subjective classification system and therefore has limited use in conveying a description or as a tool in research.

Neck Deformity

What It Classifies

The appearance of the neck for facial rejuvenation procedures.

System

See Table 4–10.

Reference

Giampapa V, Bitzos I, Ramirez O, Graneck M. Long-term results of suture suspension platysmaplasty for neck rejuvenation: a 13 year follow-up evaluation. *Aesth Plast Surg.* 2005;29(5):341–350.

Uses

Primary: Description, Diagnosis

Secondary: Treatment

Limited/none: Research, Prognosis, Etiology

Comments

Dr. Paul Oxley

This classification is designed to be used as an assessment of the neck and jowls prior to facial rejuvenation. It gives the user a standardized classification to best define the appearance of these areas.

This classification is useful for planning surgical approaches and determining how aggressive the surgeon needs to be to correct the problem. Different options exist for different levels of severity; however, this classification allows for narrowing the choices down. It has some use in research for helping to standardize preoperative states prior to different surgical options; however, it is a subjective scale and is therefore difficult to apply consistently between different users.

Table 4–10. Neck Deformity

Class	Platysmal Laxity	Submental Fat	Jowling/ Midface Laxity
1	mild	mild	none
2	mod	mod	mild
3	mod	mod	mod
4	severe	severe	severe

Source: From "Long-term results of suture suspension platysmaplasty for neck rejuvenation: a 13 year follow-up evaluation," Giampapa V, Bitzos I, Ramirez O, Graneck M. *Aesth Plast Surg.* 2005;29(5):341–350. Copyright 2005 by Springer Science and Business Media. Reprinted with kind permission from Springer Science and Business Media.

Dr. Paul L. Schnur

This classification is listed as a description of neck deformity but attempts to classify neck and midface aging deformity.

I think that any attempt to classify the aging face is fraught with inaccuracies. There are so many variations to the deformity that it is very difficult to place each patient's face into a useful classification category. To describe the changes from 1 to 4 gives a general idea as to the severity of the deformity but to try to describe each element of the deformity and place each patient into a classification level is difficult at best.

As there are so many variations to the treatment of aging face I think it is more useful to carefully describe the deformity in detail, record the changes with high-quality photography, and develop a treatment plan for the patient based on the surgeon's preference.

Platysmal Band Management

What It Classifies

Surgical correction of platysma banding.

System

See Table 4–11.

Reference

McKinney P. The management of platysma bands. *Plast Reconstr Surg.* 1996;98(6): 999–1006.

Table 4–11. Management of Platysma Banding

Bands	Visibility	Correction
I	Bands in neck barely visible	Lateral SMAS lift sufficient without midline work
II	Moderate bands visible in the neck	Require midline platysma suturing
III	Moderate bands visible in the neck	Require resection of redundant edge of muscle and midline Platysma suturing
IV	Moderate bands visible in the neck	Require midline resection and suturing as well as lateral pull.

Source: From "The management of platysma bands," McKinney P. *Plast Reconstr Surg.* 1996;98(6). Copyright 1996 by Lippincott, Williams & Wilkins. Reprinted with permission.

Uses

Primary: Description, Diagnosis, Treatment

Secondary:

Limited/none: Research, Prognosis, Etiology

Comments

Dr. Paul Oxley

The management of the neck in facial rejuvenation can be a challenging problem. It is important to define the status of the platysma and whether direct manipulation of this tissue is required. Although other authors have tried to define the anatomic structure of this muscle (see Platysma Pattern), McKinney tries to define the platysma based on the appearance in the neck and what needs to be done to correct it.

This system is designed to provide operative planning based on the clinical evaluation of the neck. It uses the natural progression of the laxity of the muscle to determine the correct surgical approach. This system, however, was designed prior to the wide spread use of suture suspension of the neck and face and should probably be revised.

Although there is some gray area between the degree of bands and he defines these subjectively, it is an easy system to use. It has little use in research except to look at the long-term outcomes for a given preoperative state.

Dr. Paul L. Schnur

This should not be considered a classification of platysma bands. Dr. McKinney describes "barely visible" and "moderately visible" platysma bands. He divides the two descriptions into four classes based on his method of treatment of the bands. There are so many variations of treatment of platysma bands and the methods change so often that to create a classification based on Dr. McKinney's approach to treatment is of no value at this time. This is not to say that Dr. McKinney is not a skilled surgeon and his treatment of the platysma bands is not an excellent method of treatment but there are many different techniques of management of platysma bands that give excellent results.

I would suggest that the extent of the bands be described in detail, high-quality photographs taken and each surgeon apply the corrective treatment that he or she deems appropriate for the deformity.

Platysmal Banding

What It Classifies

Configuration of the platysma muscle.

System

Type 1: The platysma proceeds cephalad as separate bands and only decussates for 1 to 2 cm below the edge of the mandible.

Type 2: The platysma decussates from the level of the thyroid cartilage to the mandible.

Type 3: The platysma does not decussate and remains two separate bands.

See Figure 4-3.

References

Barton FE Jr. The aging face: rejuvenation surgery and adjunctive measures. *Selected Readings in Plastic Surgery.* 1997;8(19):8.

Cordoso De Castro C. The anatomy of the platysma muscle. *Plast Reconstr Surg.* 1980;66:680.

Vistnes LM, Souther SG. The anatomical basis for common cosmetic anterior neck deformities. *Ann Plast Surg.* 1979;2:381.

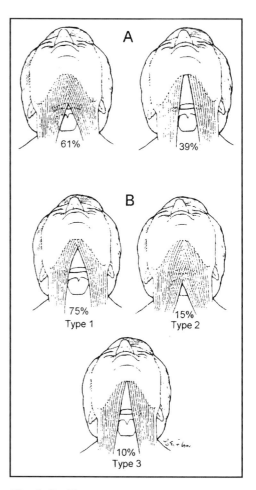

Fig 4–3. Platysma pattern. Barton FE Jr. The Aging Face: rejuvenation surgery and adjunctive measures. *Selected Readings in Plastic Surgery.* 1997; 8(19):8. Copyright 1997 by Selected Readings in Plastic Surgery. Reprinted with permission.

Uses

Primary: Description, Diagnosis, Etiology

Secondary: Research

Limited/none: Treatment, Prognosis

Comments

Dr. Paul Oxley

The platysma is an important component in the overall appearance of the neck and face. It is generally an area of focus in most facelift or neck lift procedures. In general, the greater the degree of decussation leads to less chance of pseudoherniation of the submental fat pad and platysmal banding. Understanding the different configurations of the platysma helps to determine which approach should be taken to alleviate banding.

The original description by Vistnes and Souther was based on a small study of 14 cadaveric and 21 clinical dissections. It included only two types, generally equated to types 2 and 3. Cordoso de Castro's study had a larger group and added the first type. This is a useful addition given that this can be a common finding. Treatment in each case differs.

Asian Nose

What It Classifies

Anatomic norms of the Asian nose

System

See Table 4-12.

Reference

Aung SC, Foo CL, Lee ST. Three-dimensional laser scan assessment of the Oriental nose with a new classification of Oriental nasal types. *Br J Plast Surg.* 2000;53:109.

Uses

Primary: Description, Diagnosis

Secondary: Treatment, Research

Limited/none: Prognosis, Etiology

Comments

Dr. Paul Oxley

Each ethnic group has different ideals for nasal beauty. It is important for a surgeon to understand the different types of noses seen in these groups. Some groups prefer a wider, flatter nose whereas others prize a thin, pointed one. Without this knowledge a surgeon is likely to make errors in their assessment and operative planning in cosmetic and reconstructive procedures.

This classification shows the different types of Asian nose as best assessed from a worm's eye view. The authors used 90 subjects to determine their subtypes, basing the description on tip projection and fullness, alar lobular prominence, and the slope of the lateral nasal walls.

This system, although subjective, helps the user to identify key features in the Asian nose and helps in surgical planning. It does not by itself indicate treatment, though it will help the reconstruction or repair of a nasal injury by allowing the surgeon to better understand aesthetic goals.

Table 4-12. Asian Nose

Type	Description
A	Bulbous tip
	Prominent alar lobules with broad alar base
	Wide interalar angle
	Lateral wall forms smooth and convex contour between tip and alar lobule
B	Better defined nasal tip
	Alar lobule less prominent
	Narrower interalar angle
	Lateral wall slope interrupted by indentation formed by alar groove
C	Less tip projection
	Minimal alar lobule prominence
	Lateral wall slopes in almost straight line from tip to base

Source: From "Three dimensional laser scan assessment of the Oriental nose with a new classification of Oriental nasal types," Aung SC, Foo CL, Lee ST. *Br J Plas Surg.* 2000;53, p. 109. Copyright 2000 by Lippincott, Williams & Wilkins. Reprinted with permission.

Dr. Nick Carr

This is useful as a method of thinking about the oriental nose. Specifically, each type has specific aspects to consider.

Type A is the most difficult nose as it is usually accompanied by thick skin—to gain tip shape, significant cartilage graft projection usually with columellar strut grafts and tip grafts will be required and likely also alar base resection. Type B is the easiest nose to improve aesthetically and may only require dorsal augmentation. Type C is likely to have less problems with skin thickness than Type A but will still require a combination of columellar and tip grafts to gain projection.

Boxy Nasal Tip

What It Classifies

The cause of a boxy nasal tip.

System

See Table 4-13 and Figure 4-4.

Reference

Rohrich RJ, Adams WP Jr. The boxy nasal tip: classification and management based on alar cartilage suturing techniques. *Plast Reconstr Surg.* 2001;107(7):1849-1863.

Uses

Primary: Description, Diagnosis, Treatment

Secondary:

Limited/none: Etiology, Prognosis, Research

Comments

Dr. Nick Carr and Dr. Paul Oxley

There are many anatomic parts to be considered when planning and executing

Table 4–13. Boxy Nasal Tip

Type I:	• Increased intracrural angle of divergence (>30 degrees) • Normal domal arc (4 mm or less) manifesting as tip defining points
Type II:	• Normal angle of divergence (<30 degrees) • Widened domal arc (>4 mm) • Increased angulation of domes of the lower lateral cartilage
Type III:	• Increased angle of divergence • Widened crural domal arc (4 mm or more)

Source: From "The boxy nasal tip: classification and management based on alar cartilage suturing techniques," Rohrich RJ, Adams WP Jr. *Plast Reconstr Surg.* 2001;107(7), pp. 1849–1863. Copyright 2001 by Lippincott, Williams & Wilkins. Reprinted with permission.

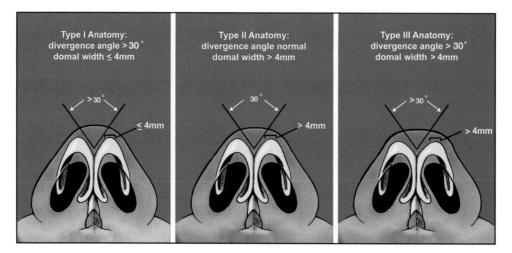

Fig 4–4. Boxy nasal tip. Rohrich RJ, Adams WP Jr. The boxy nasal tip: classification and management based on alar cartilage suturing techniques. *Plast Reconstr Surg.* 2001;107(7):1849–1863. Copyright 2001 by Lippincott, Williams & Wilkins. Reprinted with permission.

a successful rhinoplasty. A common preoperative concern by patients is the boxy nasal tip. This is a broad, rectangular shape of the tip best appreciated on basal view (Fig 4-5). This appearance can be caused by the anatomic variation of two elements: domal arc and intracrural angle. Domal arc is the distance or width of one dome. The angle of divergence is the measured angle between medial crura as they extend toward their respective domes. It is imperative that a surgeon evaluate the cause of the problem before attempting correction.

The authors help identify the cause of the problem and relate it to surgical correction using an open rhinoplasty technique. The system is based as much on intraoperative analysis as preoperative findings. Once determined, the surgical options are included in an algorithm in the original article using three nasal tip sutures

This is a very useful classification as it not only describes the anatomic variations but also offers alternatives for surgical management. It is easily understood and utilized.

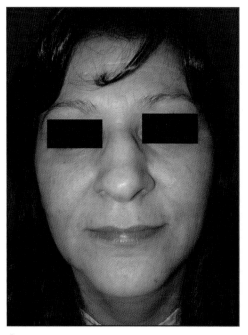
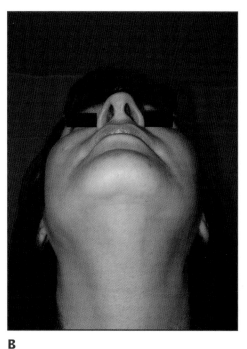

A   **B**

Fig 4–5A and B. Boxy nasal tip.

Hispanic Rhinoplasty

What It Classifies

Anatomic deformity seen in the Hispanic rhinoplasty patient.

System

Type I: High radix, a high dorsum, and a nearly normal tip.
  AKA: Castilian nose

Type II: Low radix, a normal dorsum, and a dependent tip.
  AKA: Mexican American nose

Type III: Broad base, thick skin, and a wide tip deformity.
  AKA: Mestizo nose

Type IV: Predominant black features
  AKA: Creole nose

Reference

Daniel RK. Hispanic rhinoplasty in the United States, with emphasis on the Mexican American nose. *Plast Reconstr Surg.* 2003;112(1):244-256.

Uses

Primary: Description, Treatment

Secondary:

Limited/none: Etiology, Diagnosis, Prognosis, Research

Comments

Dr. Paul Oxley

Aesthetic surgery strives to make a facial feature more attractive to the individual patient. The surgeon's job is to determine what the patient is looking for and how best to create that change. When dealing with non-Caucasian patients it is important to understand the anatomic variation seen in that population and the ethnic norms that are thought to be attractive or ideal.

This classification was developed following a limited review of only 25 patients, however. Three groups were readily apparent, and the fourth group was added based on a group of patients known to exist, none of which were in this study. The classification is based on the anatomic variation and not the ethnic origin of the patient. Where possible, the author correlated these with historical terms associated with certain appearances. The original paper also offers a treatment algorithm for each variant.

The author attempted to separate nasal appearance from the patient's origin but reverts back to using those regional terms. Although the classification devides this population into four different nasal types, it does little more than illustrate the fact that differences exist and that appropriate surgical approaches must be taken.

Dr. Paul L. Schnur

I think that classification of noses by ethnic groups is fraught with significant limitations and political incorrectness. A classification of nasal types into Caucasian, Asian, and African might have some descriptive value. Most surgeons use this scheme without even thinking of it as a classification.

There are few patients today with pure ethnic lineage. This is true for Hispanics who may be pure Spanish or a mixture of Europeans and American Indians. As American Indians have Asian lineage, this adds more variations to the group of people referred to as Hispanic.

A classification of nasal types by ethnicity might help to illustrate the fact that differences exist and a different surgical approach need be considered for each nasal type. The surgeon is best served by a careful evaluation of the anatomic variations of each nose. This should be recorded by careful description and quality photography. The surgeon should then use his or her skills to apply the proper modification to each anatomic variation that needs correction to give the patient the result that they desire.

Nasal Tip Variations

What It Classifies

Intrinsic differences in lower lateral cartilage anatomy leading to nasal tip asymmetry.

System

See Table 4–14 and Figure 4-6.

Reference

Rohrich RJ, Griffin JR. Correction of intrinsic nasal tip asymmetries in primary rhinoplasty. *Plast Reconstr Surg.* 2003;112(6): 1699-1712.

Uses

Primary: Diagnosis, Etiology, Research, Description

Secondary: Treatment

Limited/none: Prognosis

Comments

Dr. Paul Oxley

Nasal deviation is one of the more common reasons for people seeking aesthetic rhinoplasty surgery. Whether this is due to septal deviation, dorsal deviation, or tip asymmetry, many different surgical approaches exist. Each component needs to be addressed separately in a comprehensive surgical plan.

Tip asymmetry is a very common problem of varying degrees. It is normally perceived as abnormal dome or tip defining points, regardless of the underlying cause. This visibly is one dome overprojecting or a variable relationship between each dome and the midline. Although

Table 4–14. Nasal Tip Variation

Type	Pattern
I	One convex medial and middle crus paired with a contralateral concave medial crus • Convex side usually over projects the concave side • Overprojecting concave side also possible
II	Medial crura different lengths • Longer side over projects
III	Unilateral dome over projects its partner • Less projecting middle crus is splayed away from other dome
IV	Combination of above

Source: From "Correction of intrinsic nasal tip asymmetries in primary rhinoplasty," Rohrich RJ, Griffin JR. *Plast Reconstr Surg.* 2003;112(6), pp. 1699–1712. Copyright 2003 by Lippincott, Williams & Wilkins. Reprinted with permission.

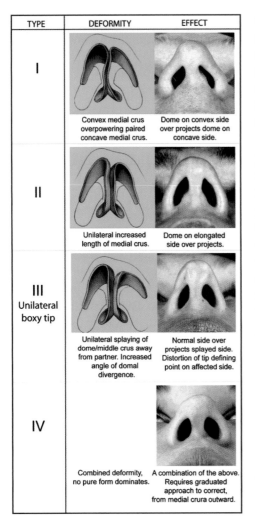

TYPE	DEFORMITY	EFFECT
I	Convex medial crus overpowering paired concave medial crus.	Dome on convex side over projects dome on concave side.
II	Unilateral increased length of medial crus.	Dome on elongated side over projects.
III Unilateral boxy tip	Unilateral splaying of dome/middle crus away from partner. Increased angle of domal divergence.	Normal side over projects splayed side. Distortion of tip defining point on affected side.
IV	Combined deformity, no pure form dominates.	A combination of the above. Requires graduated approach to correct, from medial crura outward.

Fig 4–6. Nasal tip variations. Rohrich RJ, Griffin JR. Correction of intrinsic nasal tip asymmetries in primary rhinoplasty. *Plast Reconstr Surg.* 2003; 112(6):1699–1712. Copyright 2003 by Lippincott, Williams & Wilkins. Reprinted with permission.

many of these can be identified preoperatively, it is important for the surgeon to be able to adjust the operative plan based on intraoperative findings.

Rohrich and Griffin have presented a simplified classification system of intrinsic nasal tip asymmetries and offer proposed methods of correction in their article. They note the three pure types and one combined type where no one abnormality dominates. Some noses may have two pure types thus necessitating the combined classification.

This system, as with most of those presented by Rohrich, is simple and easily applied. It takes a single clinical problem, isolates it from other contributing pathology (eg, deviated nasal dorsum), and determines the anatomic basis for the condition. It can be applied to any population and is easily reproduced. As any condition that has one aspect overprojecting versus another, treatment can always be simplified into three approaches: Taking one side forward, one back, or having both meet in between. For that reason this classification does not implicitly direct treatment and each individual's concerns and aesthetic principles must be taken into account.

Dr. Oscar M. Ramirez

This article is an attempt to organize the different intrinsic nasal tip variations in a classification system that can be used for diagnosis, surgical planning, execution of the operative techniques to correct these deformities, and for postoperative evaluation. This classification is based on the shape and length of the medial and middle crus. However, it does not include the influence of the lateral crus or the supratip deformity on the deformity of the nasal tip. Tip definition to the aesthetic judgment of patients and surgeons will need to address the influence of the other components as well. Their suggested method of surgical correction is worthwhile to consider.

Nasal L-Strut Fractures

What It Classifies

Rare types and treatment options for fractures of the L-strut in Rhinoplasty.

System

See Table 4-15 and Figure 4-7.

Reference

Gunter JP, Cochran CS. Management of intraoperative fractures of the nasal septal "L-Strut": percutaneous Kirschner wire fixation. *Plast Reconstr Surg.* 2006;117(2): 395-402.

Uses

Primary: Description, Diagnosis, Treatment

Secondary: Research

Limited/none: Prognosis, Etiology

Comments

Dr. Paul Oxley

The dorsal L-strut is created during rhinoplasty when septal cartilage is harvested for other areas in the nose. The area where the cartilaginous septum joins the perpendicular plate of the ethmoid is susceptible to overresection and when this happens a saddle nose deformity can be created. Intraoperative fractures of this strut are rare.

The authors present a classification based on 17 of 1,372 rhinoplasties in which an L-strut fracture occured. They present a K-wire fixation method as the treatment of choice for these fractures. Briefly, this includes the use of spreader grafts and/or percutaneous K-wire fixation. More details on this technique can be found in the original article. The system classifies the type and location of the fractures seen in both primary and secondary rhinoplasty.

This classification system will be rarely used as this is a very uncommon

Table 4–15. Nasal L-Strut Fracture

Type	Pattern
I	Fracture near mid portion of the cartilaginous segment of the L-strut – segment easily accessed via open approach
II	Fracture occurs cephalad to the caudal end of the nasal bones
III	Fracture occurs at or caudal to the edge of the nasal bones – difficult to access even with open approach

Source: From "Management of intraoperative fractures of the nasal septal "L-Strut": percutaneous Kirschner wire fixation," Gunter JP, Cochran CS, *Plast Reconstr Surg.* 2006;117(2), pp. 395–402. Copyright 2006 by Lippincott, Williams & Wilkins. Reprinted with permission.

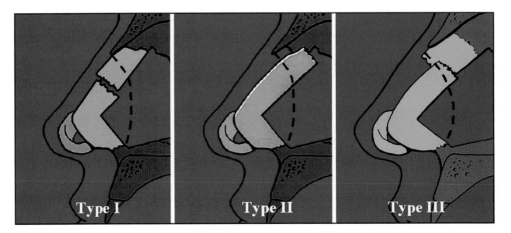

Fig 4–7. Nasal L-strut fractures. Gunter JP, Cochran CS. Management of intraoperative fractures of the nasal septal "L-Strut": percutaneous Kirschner wire fixation. *Plast Reconstr Surg.* 2006;117(2):395–402. Copyright 2006 by Lippincott, Williams & Wilkins. Reprinted with permission.

complication. This system will allow surgeons faced with this problem to understand the condition more clearly and give them confidence in treating the fracture.

The cause is usually due to overresection and therefore this system does not differentiate etiology.

Subperiosteal Facial Rejuvenation Techniques

What It Classifies

Increasing degree of subperiosteal dissection for facial rejuvenation.

System

See Table 4-16 and Figure 4-8.

Reference

Ramirez OM. Classification of facial rejuvenation techniques based on subperiosteal approach and ancillary procedures. *Plast Reconstr Surg.* 1996;97(1):45-55.

Uses

Primary: Treatment, Description

Secondary: Research, Diagnosis

Limited/none: Prognosis, Etiology

Comments

Dr. Paul Oxley

This classification was developed by Ramirez to help simplify the preoperative planning and documentation of a patient undergoing facial rejuvenation. In so doing, he hoped to make the surgical approach more easily understood by both the surgeon and the OR staff. It can also be used to help determine which procedures work better in both the short and long term for a given aesthetic problem. Ramirez allows for other techniques to be added to this classification as they are developed. He also credits the surgeons who developed the techniques.

This classification is useful for residents or surgeons early in their practice to understand the different types of facial rejuvenation and how they compare with each other. The original paper has diagrams comparing the various techniques in a given type, which help illustrate their differences.

It is limited in that it does not help the surgeon decide which approach is best suited for each patient, as there are no long-term studies looking at specific starting points.

Dr. Oscar M. Ramirez

The subperiosteal facelift of the upper and mid face described by Paul Tessier in the late 1970s and early 1980s was a straightforward operation. However, the addition of more extensive dissection on the subperiosteal plane, the combination of planes of dissection, and location of the incisions made the procedures more complex. The addition of endoscopic and biplanar techniques made the description and understanding of the complexity of the operations even more difficult.

This classification system is an excellent aid to differentiate the different variations of the subperiosteal forehead and facelift techniques and will allow more appropriate comparisons of the postoperative results obtained with one technique versus another. It will also be an excellent tool for preoperative planning and informed consent to patients.

Table 4–16. Subperiosteal Facial Rejuvenation Techniques

Subperiosteal Brow Lift and Upper Face Rejuvenation

Type I: Open (skin excision)
    A. Total subperiosteal, bicoronal (Ramirez)
    B. Subgaleal/subperiosteal bicoronal (Tessier)
    C. Classic subgaleal, limited subperiosteal
    D. Anterior hairline or modification

Type II: Full endoscopic (no skin excision)
    A. Total subperiosteal (Ramirez)
    B. Subgaleal/subperiosteal (Vasconez)
    C. Subgaleal/subperiosteal (Isse)
    D. Temporal/superolateral orbital lift (Ramirez)
    E. Procerus/corrugator ablation, frontal approach (Hamas)
    F. Procerus/corrugator ablation, temporal approach (Liang)

Type III: Biplanar (combined, semiopen, endoscopic-assisted, variable skin excision)
    A. Total biplanar (Ramirez)
    B. Anterior hairline, variable temporal extension (Ramirez)
    C. Anterior frontal hairline only (Daniel)
    D. Temporal lift only (Ramirez)

Subperiosteal Face Lift

Type IV: Open (skin excision)
    A. Extended subperiosteal/subfascial lift (Ramirez, Maillard, Musolas)
    B. Forhead-periorbtal-cheek lift (Tessier, Krastinova, Psillakis, Dempsey)
    C. Without preauricular incisions (Fuente del Campo)
    D. Temporofacial, no central forehead lift (Ramirez)

Type V: Full endoscopic (no skin excision)
    A. Total face (Ramirez)
    B. Endoforehead-endomidface (Ramirez)
    C. Endo/temporomidface, no central forehead (Ramirez)
    D. Endo/forehead-periorbital-cheek lift (Ramirez)

Type VI: Biplanar (combined, semiopen, endoscopic-assisted, variable skin excision)
    A. Total biplanar continuous (Ramirez)
    B. Total biplanar discontinuous (Ramirez)
    C. Endoforehead-biplanar face (Ramirez)
    D. Biplanar forehead-endoface lift (Ramirez)
    E. Biplanar face, no forehead lift (Ramirez)
    F. Endoforehead-biplanar face without preauricular incisions (Fuente del Campo)

Source: From "Classification of facial rejuvenation techniques based on subperiosteal approach and ancillary procedures," Ramirez OM, *Plast Reconstr Surg.* 1996;97(1), pp.45–55. Copyright 1996 by Lippincott, Williams & Wilkins. Reprinted with permission.

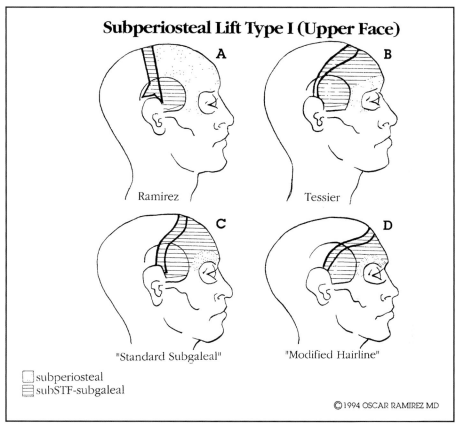

A

Fig 4–8. Subperiosteal facial rejuvenation techniques. Ramirez OM. Classification of facial rejuvenation techniques based on subperiosteal approach and ancillary procedures. *Plast Reconstr Surg.* 1996;97(1): 45–55. Copyright 1996 by Lippincott, Williams & Wilkins. Reprinted with permission. *continues*

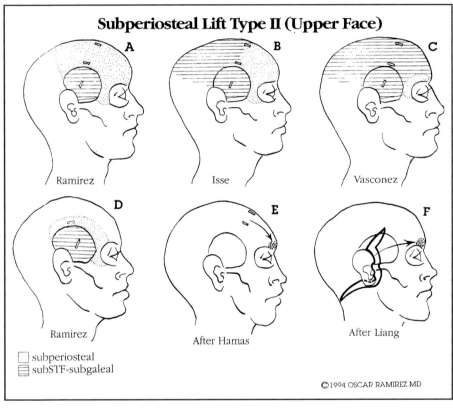

Subperiosteal Lift Type II (Upper Face)

A Ramirez

B Isse

C Vasconez

D Ramirez

E After Hamas

F After Liang

 subperiosteal
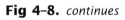 subSTF-subgaleal

©1994 OSCAR RAMIREZ MD

B

Fig 4–8. *continues*

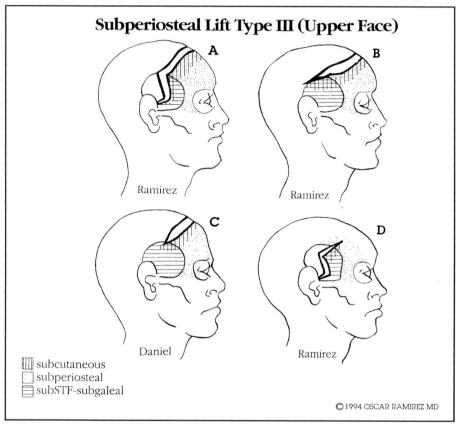

Subperiosteal Lift Type III (Upper Face)

A

Ramirez

B

Ramirez

C

Daniel

D

Ramirez

 subcutaneous
subperiosteal
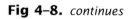 subSTF-subgaleal

© 1994 OSCAR RAMIREZ MD

C

Fig 4–8. *continues*

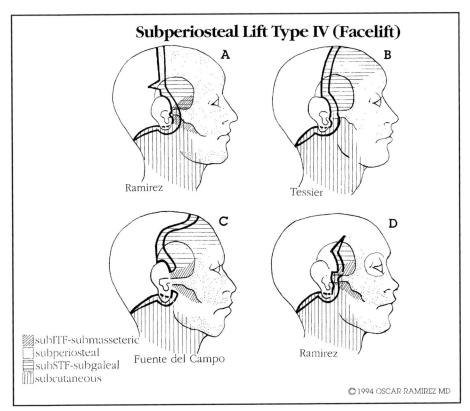

Subperiosteal Lift Type IV (Facelift)

A — Ramirez

B — Tessier

C — Fuente del Campo

D — Ramirez

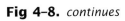 subITF-submasseteric
subperiosteal
subSTF-subgaleal
subcutaneous

© 1994 OSCAR RAMIREZ MD

D

Fig 4–8. *continues*

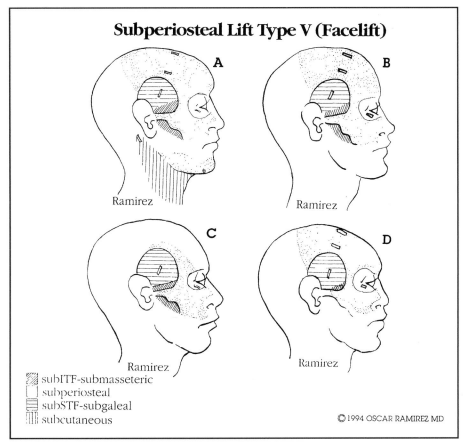

Subperiosteal Lift Type V (Facelift)

A

B

Ramirez

Ramirez

C

D

Ramirez

Ramirez

subITF-submasseteric
subperiosteal
subSTF-subgaleal
subcutaneous

© 1994 OSCAR RAMIREZ MD

E

Fig 4–8. *continues*

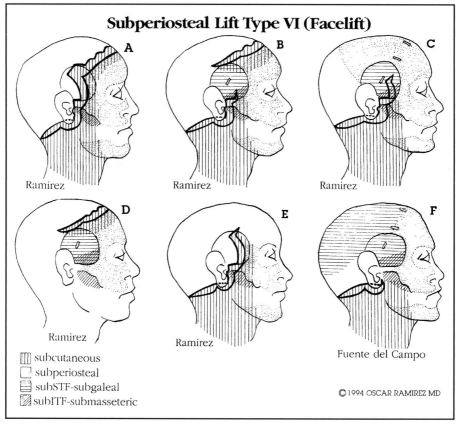

Subperiosteal Lift Type VI (Facelift)

A — Ramirez

B — Ramirez

C — Ramirez

D — Ramirez

E — Ramirez

F — Fuente del Campo

▥ subcutaneous
☐ subperiosteal
▤ subSTF-subgaleal
▨ subITF-submasseteric

©1994 OSCAR RAMIREZ MD

F

Fig 4–8. *continued*

Chapter 5

DESCRIPTIVE

Angle Classification

What It Classifies

Dental occlusion and relationships: the position of upper versus the lower jaw using specific teeth as reference points.

System

I: (neutroocclusion) mesiobuccal cusp of maxillary 1st molar articulates within the buccal groove of the lower first molar

II: (malocclusion) mesiobuccal cusp of maxillary 1st molar articulates anterior to the buccal groove of the lower first molar. Lower dentition is posterior relative to upper.

   IIa: labially flared upper incisors

   IIb: lingual flaring of upper incisors

III: (malocclusion) mesiobuccal cusp of maxillary 1st molar articulates posterior to the buccal groove of the lower first molar. Lower dentition is anterior relative to upper.

See Figure 5-1.

References

Angle EH. *Treatment of Malocclusion of the Teeth and Fractures of the Maxillae. Angle's System.* Philadelphia, Pa: SS White Publications; 1898.

Manson PN. Facial fractures. In: Aston SJ, Beasley RW, Thorne CHM, eds. *Grabb and Smith's Plastic Surgery.* 5th ed. Philadelphia, Pa: Lippincott-Raven Publishers; 1997:386.

Uses

Primary: Description, Diagnosis

Secondary: Treatment, Research, Prognosis

Limited/none: Etiology

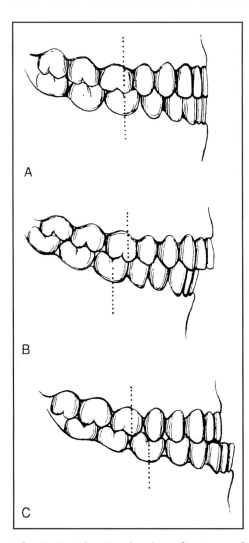

Fig 5–1. The Angle classification of occlusion. **A.** Class I, normal occlusion. **B.** Class II, retroocclusion or mandibular deficiency. **C.** Class III, prognathic occlusion (maxillary deficiency or mandibular access). The key relationships to be discerned are the relationship of the first molar teeth, the cuspid and incisor teeth. Angle. Manson PN, Facial fractures. In: Aston SJ, Beasley RW, Thorne CHM, eds, *Grabb and Smith's Plastic Surgery*, 5th ed. Philadelphia, Pa: Lippincott-Raven Publishers; 1997:386. Copyright 1997 by Lippincott, Williams & Wilkins. Reprinted with permission.

Comments

Dr. Paul Oxley

This is an extensively used classification system from the "father" of orthodontics. It is very useful in description and diagnosis of malocclusion due to either congenital or acquired conditions. The treatment depends largely on the degree of malocclusion and the presence or absence of other signs and symptoms. Prognosis depends on degree of malocclusion and underlying disease process.

The Angle classification is used for adult dentition; it is not applicable in early childhood when the deciduous teeth are present. It is often used for congenital conditions, such as retrognathia to help determine types of osteotomies that might be of use in correcting the condition. The other major use is in trauma when resetting normal occlusion after a mandibular or Le Fort fracture.

Dr. David Naysmith

Edward H Angle introduced his classification of occlusion in 1899 and based it on the relationship of the upper and lower first permanent molars. The three broad classes are: Class I (neutroclusion), Class II (distoclusion), and Class III (mesioclusion). He further divided Class II into Division 1 and Division 2. The "key to occlusion" in his classification is the mesiobuccal cusp of the upper first molar and its relationship to the lower first molar. If the lower mesiobuccal groove sits under the mesiobuccal cusp of the upper first molar it is an Angle Class I, which he described as a normal occlusion. A mesiobuccal groove of the lower molar that is posterior (distal) to the mesiobuccal cusp of the upper molar defines a Class II relationship, that is, the lower arch is distal or posterior to the upper arch. The Class II Division 1 is the typical buck toothed appearance with the maxillary incisors flared out and usually a V-shaped upper arch and deep overbite and significant overjet (but, that is the topic of another classification), and the Class II Division 2 has the upper laterals flared anteriorly and the central incisors tipped lingually. When the mesiobuccal groove of the lower molar is anterior (mesial) to the mesiobuccal cusp of the upper molar a Class III relationship is described with the usual prognathic appearance of the individual and the anterior teeth usually in complete crossbite and the lower incisors tipped lingually.

Early criticism of Angle's classification focused on the fact that facial profiles were not always predictable based on the dental relationships, as evident by a Class I occlusion in the patient with bimaxillary protrusion. As well, although the dental classification usually predicts the relationship of the basal bone of the jaws this is not always the case and thus the importance of cephalometric analysis.

The entire system of classification of course depends on some knowledge of dental anatomy (usually gained by sitting for hours with a small knife in one hand and a piece of chalk in the other whittling out giant facsimiles of human teeth so that once all the nooks and crannies of various molars, premolars, canines, and incisors have been perfected, the neophyte dental student can graduate to a high-speed drill and the enamel of some poor unsuspecting dental clinic patient. All in all, having been through it myself, an endeavor best described as "the rape of time!"). Anything that is closer to the midline of the dental arch is deemed to be mesial (what most of us would call anterior) and anything in the arch closer to the back of the mouth is distal (posterior to the unwashed). One then needs to know that the upper first molar has a mesiobuccal cusp and a distobuccal cusp and that the lower first molar a mesiobuccal groove and a distobuccal groove (which of course means the lower first molar has three buccal cusps—but really, who cares?).

From my point of view as a plastic surgeon the usefulness of Angle's classification is limited. Like many classifications it is simply a means of communication in describing what it is that we see. The particular Classes are not in any way what might be called "goals of a treatment plan" for either trauma surgery or orthognathic surgery. I well remember one of my favorite staffmen asking if I thought it was a good idea to take the opportunity to put the teeth into Class I occlusion when treating a fractured mandible. The correct answer is, of course, "only if the wear facets indicate that the teeth were in Class I relationship before the fracture occurred." It is important to note that once teeth have been extracted (for decay or orthodontic reasons) or if significant decay has diminished the anteroposterior dimension of the teeth, that the Angle classification will change and not be a reflection of the basal bone relationships. Having said that, I think it is important for surgeons to be aware of the classification for no other reason than it makes it easier to communicate with our dental colleagues while sharing patient care. Orthodontists will frequently refer to intermaxillary wires or elastics as Class II or Class III traction if we are trying to guide the occlusion in a specific fashion and it is important for surgeons to understand the implications of such treatment.

Given a choice between learning the Angle classification and learning how to read wear facets on teeth, choose the latter.

Malar Hypoplasia

What It Classifies

The anatomic causes of irregularities in cheek contour.

AKA

Binder's Classification of Malar Hypoplasia

System

I. Malar deficiency
II. Submalar deficiency
III. Severe prominence with severe submalar hollow
IV. Malar and submalar hypoplasia
V. Tear trough deformity

References

Binder WJ. Submalar augmentation: a procedure to enhance rhytidectomy. *Ann Plast Surg.* 1990;24(3):200–212.
Binder WJ, Kaye A. Reconstruction of post-traumatic and congenital facial deformities with three-dimensional computer assisted custom designed implants. *Plast Reconstr Surg.* 1994;94(6):775–785.

Uses

Primary: Etiology, Description, Treatment

Secondary: Diagnosis

Limited/none: Research, Prognosis

Comments

Dr. Paul Oxley

Midfacial aging and the appearance of the zygomatic region are difficult areas for the reconstructive and aesthetic surgeon. As in many areas of the face, to properly treat the problem, an understanding of normal and abnormal appearances is essential. Recently there has been an interest by surgeons like Binder to classify the normal anatomy from an aesthetic point of view and the sequelae of aging.

Binder's classification is relatively new and is not yet widely used. It will likely gain wider use in time. This system breaks down malar irregularities in an orderly and easily followed manner. However, it does not describe the degree of abnormality nor does it address uniformly the boney versus soft tissue issues. For example, the lack of projection of a malar eminence may be due to ptosis of the malar fat pad into a submalar hollow. Nevertheless, this system trains the user to focus on this very important area of the face. Treatment can be determined from the identified problem in most cases.

Ear Lobe Ptosis

What It Classifies

Degree of ptosis of the ear lobe.

System

See Table 5–1.

References

Mowlavi A, Meldrum DG, Wilhelmi BJ, Ghavami A, Zook EG. The aesthetic earlobe: classification of lobule ptosis on the basis of a survey of North American Caucasians. *Plast Reconstr Surg.* 2003;112(1):266–272.

Mowlavi A, Meldrum DG, Wilhelmi BJ, Zook EG. Incidence of earlobe ptosis and pseudoptosis in patients seeking facial rejuvenation surgery and effects of aging. *Plast Reconstr Surg.* 2004;113(2):712–717.

Uses

Primary: Description

Secondary: Research, Treatment

Limited/none: Diagnosis, Prognosis, Etiology

Table 5–1. Earlobe Ptosis

Ptosis Grade	Otobasion Inferius to Subaurale Distance (mm)
0	0
I	1–5
II	6–10
III	11–15
IV	16–20
V	>20

Pseudoptosis	Intertragal Notch to Otobasion Inferius Distance
Normal	Less than or equal to 15 mm
Abnormal	Greater than 15 mm

Source: From "Incidence of earlobe ptosis and pseudoptosis in patients seeking facial rejuvenation surgery and effects of aging," Mowlavi A, Meldrum DG, Wilhelmi BJ, Zook EG, *Plast Reconstr Surg.* 2004;113(2):712–717. Copyright 2004 by Lippincott, Williams & Wilkins. Reprinted with permission.

Comments

Dr. Paul Oxley

The authors of this paper looked at the aesthetic earlobe and devised a classification system based on the distance from the otobasion inferius to the subaurale point, or in other words, the free caudal segment. They believe that by defining the degree of ptosis, either present or desired, reconstructive and cosmetic revision can be better planned and performed. The authors note that this measurement is superior to the intertragal notch to otobasion inferius distance due to the latter's less reliable measurement and its poorer correlation to aesthetically pleasing earlobes. Nevertheless, they used this number, however, to define the attached caudal segment, which was the defining point for the degree of pseudoptosis in a later paper. They found that males and females could be graded with the same system. Ideal ptosis was classified as Grade I.

This classification was developed for the Caucasian population and has yet to be applied to other ethnic groups. Ear lobe correction is most commonly indicated for problems with piercing—either torn or stretched lobes. As the prevalence of ear lobe stretching becomes greater, it is natural to believe that the long-term demand for corrective procedures will increase as well. This classification is a very precise, easily reproducible system that is best used for describing the condition and perhaps to be used in research into the procedures used to correct it.

Dr. Don Guichon

This is a classification for "splitters" rather than "lumpers." That said it has useful application for research into what the "normal" is. What I believe most valuable about this classification is that it challenges plastic surgeons to consider with an artistic sense the esthetics of the earlobe. The classification may never be used by a day-to-day plastic surgeon, but the underlying thought that has gone into this article makes it a "must read" for the developing surgeon. The concepts are novel, creative, and challenge us all to consider what is normal and what is desirable from an appearance point of view.

Jelks' Classification

What It Classifies

Position of the ocular globe versus the lower lid and malar eminence.

AKA

Jelks Vectors

System

Positive: The anterior most projection of the globe lies behind the lower eyelid margin, which lies behind the anterior projection of the malar eminence.

Neutral: The anterior most projection of the globe lies in a vertical line with the lower eyelid margin and the malar eminence.

Negative: The anterior most projection of the globe lies anterior to the lower eyelid margin, which lies anterior to the anterior projection of the malar eminence.

Reference

Note. Portions of this section were taken from "Preoperative evaluation of the blepharoplasty patient—bypassing the pitfalls," Jelks GW, Jelks EB, *Clinics in Plastic Surgery*, 1993;20(2), p. 213. Copyright 1993 by Elsevier. Reprinted with permission.

Uses

Primary: Description, Treatment

Secondary: Prognosis, Etiology

Limited/none: Research, Diagnosis

Comments

Dr. Paul Oxley

This classification is an important one to help a surgeon decide on the appropriate procedure for lower lid rejuvenation without running into the serious postoperative complications of excess scleral show or ectropion. Although many eyelid malpositions are temporary, the persistent ones can cause significant discomfort to the patient and to the surgeon.

The vector is determined on the lateral view; it is a description of the relationship between the lower lid and malar eminence, and the anterior projection of the globe. It reflects the bony and ligamentous structures around the eye and how they will compensate for lower lid blepharoplastic changes. The simplest way of looking at this is whether there is positive or negative support. For example, the positive vector shows a favorable condition for lower lid blepharoplasty due to strong bony and ligamentous support for the lid.

Dr. Luis Vasconez

An understanding of the position of the eyeball in relation to the lower lid is important. The discrepancy is obvious and most severe in cases of exophthalmus.

Presently, and in practical terms, the vectors have less clinical importance because we are doing a lesser number of isolated lower blepharoplasties. This is true, because we have a better understanding of the changes in the lower lid due to gravity and aging. As we age, the distinct skin of the lower lid descends below the infraorbital rim, whereas in youth it is above the rim. To restore the youthful position of the lower lid, one has to do a midface elevation.

Another important concept is the detection of horizontal lid laxity or vertical deficit. The former is ameliorated by tightening the lower lid with a canthoplasty or by a wedge resection of the tarsus of the lower lid. Vertical deficit is corrected by placement of so called "spacers."

I believe the concepts of laxity, vertical deficit, and our conservatism in lower lid surgery are the most important factors. Vectors should be observed, and are indicative of what one needs to do to avoid problems. Tightening the orbicularis muscle in the lower lid is another important factor.

Chapter 6

NERVE

Facial Paralysis

What It Classifies

The severity of facial palsy.

AKA

House-Brackman Classification

System

1. Normal appearance and function
2. Normal symmetry and tone at rest, slight weakness/oral asymmetry, slight or no synkenesis
3. Normal symmetry and tone at rest, obvious weakness, some synkenesis
4. Normal symmetry and tone at rest, inability to elevate brow, incomplete eye closure
5. Resting asymmetry, motion barely perceptible
6. No tone

Reference

Note. This section was taken from the article published in *Otolaryngology-Head*

Neck Surgery, 1985;93(2):146–147. House JW, Brackmann DE, "Facial nerve grading system." Copyright 1985 by Elsevier. Reprinted with permission.

Uses

Primary: Description, Treatment, Diagnosis

Secondary: Prognosis, Research

Limited/none: Etiology

Comments

Dr. Paul Oxley

This is a very good classification of severity of facial palsy. It is useful in description and has fairly strict criteria, although there is some room for subjectivity in the grading. Its role in diagnosis can be limited as it is more of a description of the disease. It does not differentiate the cause of the palsy which can be an important part of the diagnosis. Most clinicians will want to know if the cause is known, such as with trauma or tumours, or unknown, in the case of Bell's palsy.

Treatment of the condition is generally directed by the severity of the disease, though other factors such as patient age, etiology, and speed of onset must be considered. Prognosis depends as much on etiology, rapidity of onset, and time to treatment as it does on severity.

Sunderland Classification of Nerve Injury

What It Classifies

Degree of nerve injury.

System

See Table 6-1.

References

Sunderland S. *Nerves and Nerve Injuries*. 2nd ed. Edinburgh: Churchill Livingstone, 1978.

Brandt KE, Mackinnon SE. Microsurgical repair of peripheral nerves and nerve grafts. In: Aston SJ, Beasley RW, Thorne CHM, eds. *Grabb and Smith's Plastic Surgery*. 5th ed. Philadelphia, Pa: Lippincott-Raven Publishers; 1997:79.

Uses

Primary: Description, Prognosis, Diagnosis, Treatment

Secondary: Etiology, Research

Limited/none:

Table 6-1. Sunderland Nerve Injury

Degree Injury	Tinel	Recovery	Rate of Recovery	Surgery	Like
First	No	Full	Days to weeks (<12)	No	Neuropraxia
Second	Yes	Full	1mm/day	No	Axonotmesis
Third	Yes	Variable	1mm/day	Neurolysis	Axonotmesis
Fourth	Stagnant	None	None	Repair	NIC
Fifth	Stagnant	None	None	Repair	Neurotmesis
Sixth	Variable	Variable	Variable	Variable	Combined

NIC = Neuroma in Continuity.
Source: From "Microsurgical Repair of Peripheral Nerves and Nerve Grafts." Brandt KE, Mackinnon SE. In: Aston SJ, Beasley RW, Thorne CHM, eds. *Grabb and Smith's Plastic Surgery*, 5th ed. Philadelphia, Pa: Lippincott-Raven Publishers; 1997:79. Copyright 1997 by Lippincott, Williams & Wilkins. Reprinted with permission.

Comments

Dr. Paul Oxley

This classification expands on the Seddon scheme and recognizes injuries that do not fall easily into one of those groups. Seddon classified nerve injuries with three degrees as first degree (neuropraxia), second degree (axonotmesis), and third degree (neurotmesis).

The Sunderland classification is widely used, though the terms from the Seddon classification tend to be used by physicians and surgeons who do not deal with these injuries on a regular basis. Research usually depends on nerve conduction studies or electromyograms as the gold standard. MRI is replacing clinical exploration in some cases to determine physical discontinuity of the nerve itself.

The major drawback is that it often requires waiting for time to pass before exact diagnosis and classification can be assigned. This may affect final outcome in some circumstances.

The original Sunderland classification does not include the sixth degree or mixed injury state often seen in larger nerves. Mackinnon added this category to include those types of injuries.

Sunderland Classification of Neuromas

What It Classifies

Types of neuromas in injured nerves.

System

   I. Neuromas-in-continuity
     A. Spindle neuromas. Lesions in which the perineurium is not broken.
     B. Lateral neuromas. Lesions in which the perineurium of some funiculi is broken.
     C. Neuromas following nerve repair
  II. Neuromas in completely severed nerves
 III. Amputation stump neuromas

References

Note. From "Neuromas," Herndon JH, in *Operative Hand Surgery,* 3rd ed, Green DP, ed, New York, NY: Churchill Livingstone; 1993:1389. Copyright 1993 by Elsevier. Reprinted with permission.

Sunderland S. *Nerves and Nerve Injuries.* 2nd ed. Edinburgh: Churchill Livingstone; 1978.

Uses

Primary: Description, Diagnosis, Etiology

Secondary: Research

Limited/none: Treatment, Prognosis

Comments

Dr. Paul Oxley

A post-traumatic neuroma forms when a peripheral nerve is disrupted and attempts to regenerate. While regrowing it forms a ball of neural fibers rather than growing longitudinally. This ball is typically painful.

This is a descriptive classification of different neuromas that occur after trauma. It is useful as well in conveying diagnosis. Generally, however, neuromas tend to be described without using this classification. Terms such as neuroma-in-continuity and amputation stump neuroma are used in many cases, but the other terms are less utilized.

The classification has some use in research and limited to no use in determining prognosis. Treatment options are related to the type of neuroma but many options exist that are not necessarily specific to any one type. Location, patient age, and severity of symptoms play a large part in deciding treatment.

Chapter 7

RECONSTRUCTIVE

Fasciocutaneous Flaps (Cormack and Lamberty)

What It Classifies

Blood flow into fasciocutaneous flaps.

System

A: Multiple random, unnamed fasciocutaneous perforator vessels
B: Single fasciocutaneous perforator vessel with consistent presence and location (eg, scapular, parascapular)
   B modified: Type B vessel which is harvested along with its vessel of origin
C: Single deep vessel with multiple perforators feeds flap (eg, radial forearm, lateral arm)
D: Same as C with the addition of bone (osteomyofasciocutaneous)

References

Lamberty BG, Cormack GC. Fasciocutaneous flaps. *Clin Past Surg.* 1990;17(4):713–726.
Cormack GC, Lamberty BGH. A classification of fasciocutaneous flaps according to their patterns of vascularisation. *Br J Plast Surg.* 1984;37:80.
Barclay TC, Cardoso E, Sharpe DT, Crockett DJ. Repair of lower leg injuries with fasciocutaneous flaps. *Br J Plast Surg.* 1982; 35:127.
Haertsch PA. The surgical plane in the leg. *Br J Plast Surg.* 1981;35:464.
Mathes SJ, Nahai F. *Reconstructive Surgery: Principles, Anatomy, and Technique.* New York, NY, Churchill Livingstone; 1997.
Nakajima H, Minabe T, Imanishi N. Three-dimensional analysis and classification of arteries in the skin and subcutaneous adipofascial tissue by computer graphics imaging. *Plast Reconstr Surg.* 1998;102:748.
Ponten B. The fasciocutaneous flap: its use in soft tissue defects of the lower leg. *Br J Plast Surg.* 1981;34:215.

Uses

Primary: Description

Secondary: Treatment

Limited/none: Research, Diagnosis, Etiology, Prognosis

Comments

Dr. Paul Oxley

Fasciocutaneous flaps are classified using either this system or the one put forth by Mathes and Nahai. Unlike the other system, this encompasses all fasciocutaneous flaps, including ones that have an essentially random blood supply. Thus, it can be used for all local and free fasciocutaneous flaps.

With the advent of perforator flaps as workhorses of reconstructive surgery, this classification is less definitive than the Mathes and Nahai system. For example, it does not differentiate the pattern in which the dominant blood vessel or perforator supplies the flap, whether through a septum or muscle.

It still has its place in understanding different types of flaps, and is therefore more useful for the student than the practicing surgeon. It is purely a descriptive classification with little use in research or defining treatment options.

Dr. Martin Jugenburg and Dr. Andrea Pusic

Fasciocutaneous flaps have gained tremendous popularity because of their ease of elevation, less bulk, high reliability, and easier transfer than either muscle or musculocutaneous flaps. Additionally, unlike muscle flaps, they come without subsequent functional impairment

Ponten in 1981 first described skin flap elevation based on the deep fascial vascular plexus. More was then written on this subject by Haertsch and Barclay et al. Schaefer then went on to describe three types of vascular supplies to these flaps: perforating arteries, subcutaneous arteries, and subfascial arteries. Cormack and Lamberty subsequently created a more specific classification system. However, unlike the Mathes and Nahai classification of muscles, this classification system is not as widely utilized. Although muscle and muscle flaps are a distinct anatomic and vascular entity, whose blood supply dictates how they can be used as flaps, fasciocutaneous flaps are thought of more as angiosomes rather than distinct anatomic entities. Fasciocutaneous flaps are thus designed around known perforator vessels. Perhaps a simpler, and clinically more relevant vascular classification is the Mathes and Nahai classification of fasciocutaneous flaps which describes the path of the feeding vessels.

Cutaneous Flaps

What It Classifies

Different flap patterns and blood supplies for skin flaps.

System

See Table 7–1.

Table 7–1. Cutaneous Flaps

By Blood Supply
Random pattern
No named blood supply
Axial
Blood supply from direct, named cutaneous vessels
By Pattern (Mobilization)
Local
Rotation (Local flaps moving around a fixed point)
Rotation
Transposition
Interpolated
Advancement (Flap advancement without rotation or lateral movement)
Single pedicle
Bipedicle
Distant
Random or axial supply, move to an area separated from the donor site

Source: From Fisher J, Gingrass MK, Principles of skin flaps, in: Georgiade GS, Riefkohl R, & Levin LS, eds, *Georgiade Plastic, Maxillofacial and Reconstructive Surgery*, 3rd ed, Baltimore, Md: Williams and Wilkins, 1997:19–21. Copyright 1997 by Lippincott, Williams & Wilkins. Reprinted with permission.

Reference

Fisher J, Gingrass MK. Basic principles of skin flaps. In: Georgiade GS, Riefkohl R, & Levin LS, eds. *Georgiade Plastic, Maxillofacial and Reconstructive Surgery.* 3rd ed. Baltimore, Md: Williams and Wilkins, 1997:19–21.

Uses

Primary: Description

Secondary: Treatment, Research

Limited/none: Etiology, Diagnosis, Prognosis

Comments

Dr. Paul Oxley

Almost every procedure plastic surgeons do is related to one type of flap or another. Whether it is a small bilobed flap, a cleft lip repair, a free flap, or a face lift, they all can be classified at their basic most level using this type of system. The system put forth by Fisher and Gingrass is one of the easiest to understand when trying to learn how flaps work. For that reason it is of most use to the student or resident, though it also touches on the day-to-day practice of all plastic surgeons.

This system is a descriptive classification of the blood supply and mobilization of cutaneous flaps. For the student it is essential to be able to look at any flap and be able to place it within this system. Regardless of the components of the flap they can all be described by one of the above options. For any given defect, one can scan through the myriad options available, understand these principles, and help direct treatment choices for that defect.

Dr. Charles Snelling

Under the random pattern heading in this classification no named blood supply is provided but, in fact, the blood supply is the subdermal and subcapillary plexi. These plexi, although not having a specific name, do refer to a well-recognized system of blood vessels.

Under pattern mobilization and local flaps there is the subclassification of rotation flap. I believe in this context it refers to a flap which is of sufficient size so that when it rotates into a defect there is still enough flap to close the donor site. Transposition flap refers to the fact that when the flap is swiveled about its rotation point it is of such a size that the defect created cannot be closed by redistributing the flap itself but requires a skin graft or a second flap. For example, a transposition with a second flap may be a Z-plasty or a Limberg flap. Interpolated is best exemplified by the bilobe flap.

Under distant flaps it should be stressed that the base of the flap will subsequently be separated from its donor site once neocirculation has been established.

Finally, there are two other aspects that need to be considered. One is the cutaneous flap that also contains other structures such as a myocutaneous flap. And the other would be flaps requiring either a delay or multiple stages to achieve their desired result.

Dr. Colleen McCarthy

This classification system categorizes cutaneous flaps in the broadest sense. It is a system that differentiates by blood supply and method of mobilization, but does not further classify each flap within each group. It provides, however, a simple, straightforward way to think about skin flaps, how they are designed, and how they can be used to reconstruct cutaneous defects. It is easy to interpret and easy to use. Although some may think this classification system outdated or "too simple," such a schema can be invaluable when teaching plastic surgical principles to beginner surgeons and/or when a complex wound closure forces even the expert surgeon to "go back to basics."

Fasciocutaneous Flaps

What It Classifies

Flap composition, vascular anatomy, and utilization.

System

By vascular anatomy

Axial pattern flap

Meso flap or septocutaneous flap

Neurocutaneous flap

By utilization

Proximally or distally based island pedicled flaps

Peninsular flaps with a proximal or a distal hinge

Free vascularized flaps

By component tissues of the flap

Fascial flap

Vascularized fat flap

Cutaneous flap

Fasciocutaneous flap

Reference

Masquelet A, Romano MC. Principles of fasciocutaneous flaps. In: Georgiade GS, Riefkohl R, & Levin LS, eds. *Georgiade Plastic, Maxillofacial and Reconstructive Surgery*. 3rd ed. Baltimore, Md: Williams and Wilkins, 1997:19–21.

Uses

Primary: Description

Secondary: Treatment, Research

Limited/none: Diagnosis, Prognosis, Etiology

Comments

Dr. Paul Oxley

This system is a basic classification of flaps and outlines their major characteristics. It is descriptive, is best used to understand different flaps, and is especially useful as a learning tool. It is an important system for a student to understand as it divides each flap into its separate components. Through this understanding and experience with different flaps, a student will be better able to determine which flaps are best suited for a given problem.

This classification system is not designed to convey any sort of diagnosis or prognosis. As a research tool it may be useful in defining a flap that is being studied but has little value by itself.

Dr. Colleen McCarthy

There are numerous ways to classify fasiocutaneous flaps. Schaefer et al classified the vascular supplies to these flaps as: perforating arteries, subcutaneous arteries, and subfascial arteries. Cormack and Lamberty subsequently created a more specific classification system based on blood flow into a fasciocutaneous flap. Mathes and Nahai have also further defined various types of fasciocutaneous flaps.

No one classification system is considered the "gold standard" here. Masquelet et al system is ambitious in that it attempts to classify the composition, vascular anatomy, and utilization of various fasciocutaneous flaps. It is this author's opinion, however, that what is left is a schema of limited clinical utility.

Hypopharynx Defect

What It Classifies

The extent of hypopharyx defects following resection and suggestions for surgical correction of each.

System

See Table 7–2.

Reference

Disa JJ, Pusic AL, Hidalgo DA, Cordeiro PG. Microvascular reconstruction of the hypopharynx: defect classification, treatment algorithm, and functional outcome based on 165 consecutive cases. *Plast Reconstr Surg.* 2003;111(2):652–660.

Uses

Primary: Description, Treatment

Secondary: Research

Limited/none: Etiology, Diagnosis, Prognosis

Comments

Dr. Paul Oxley

Resection of the hypopharynx for oncologic clearance can result in significantly

Table 7–2. Hypopharynx Defects

Type	Defect	Closure
0	small	Closed directly with primary closure
I	<50% circumference	Fasciocutaneous flap
II	>50% circumference	Free jejunum
III	extensive longitudinal	Rectus abdominis myocutaneous flap
IV	include thoracic esophagus	Gastric pull-up

Source: From "Microvascular reconstruction of the hypopharynx: defect classification, treatment algorithm, and functional outcome based on 165 consecutive cases," Disa JJ, Pusic AL, Hidalgo DA, Cordeiro PG, *Plast Reconstr Surg.* 2003;111(2):652–660. Copyright 2003 by Lippincott, Williams & Wilkins. Reprinted with permission.

different defects. This ranges from small, easily closed defects up to those requiring free flaps or gastric pull-up procedures. The defects can be very complex including parts of the floor of the mouth, tongue, esophagus, and larynx, as well as the oral and nasal pharynx. Each resected area has certain functions that need to be reconstructed to provide the best outcome for these patients.

This classification was derived from operations on 165 patients. The authors analyzed the size of the defect and offer the appropriate surgical option chosen by their group. The classification they present includes Types I to III and they add Types 0 and IV as natural extensions not specifically reviewed in the study. They focus on determining the three intermediate types as these pose the greatest surgical decision-making challenge and require microsurgical reconstruction.

The classification is limited in its wider application as it looks primarily at circumferential or longitudinal defects in the hypopharynx requiring microvascular reconstruction and does not comment on the extent of other involvement (eg, larynx). By itself it does not convey diagnosis or prognosis. It is very useful to help intraoperative decision making following ablation of a tumour.

Dr. Martin Jugenburg and Dr. Andrea Pusic

The reconstructive surgeon can analyze the defect and a simple rule of thumb can be applied. Defects less than 50% circumference of the hypopharynx are best reconstructed with a fasciocutaneous flap. If greater than 50% of the circumference, reconstruction is best performed with a free jejunum flap. For large longitudinal defects, the rectus flap is preferred.

The descriptive value of this classification is excellent, as it clearly communicates the extent of the defect. For operative decision-making purposes, this classification system then helps to determine the most appropriate method of reconstruction.

Dr. Fu-Chan Wei and Dr. Perry Liu

This classification for hypopharynx defects seems reasonable, easy to interpret, and easy to utilize. The closure of these defects appears to be outdated. For type I–II defects, ALT closure has probably replaced the listed options as the preferred reconstructive modality. It provides superior results in terms of phonation and bacterial translocation rates. Jejunal hypopharynx reconstructions may have less leakage because mucosa to mucosa healing is better than mucosa to skin healing. However, the speech associated with free jejunal flaps is very wet and much harder to comprehend. Although gastric pull-up is a viable and often used technique for reconstructing Type IV defects, colonic interposition graft is another viable alternative. Hypopharyngeal defects could also be closed using supraclavicular pedicled or free flaps. Although not a primary option, it is a good backup option.

Fasciocutaneous Flaps (Mathes and Nahai)

What It Classifies

Blood flow into fasciocutaneous flaps.

System

A: Subcutaneous pedicle (eg, temperoparietal)
B: Fasciocutaneous perforators (eg, radial forearm)
C: Musculocutaneous perforators (eg, TRAM, DIEP)

See Figure 7–1.

Reference

Mathes SJ, Nahai F. Flap selection: analysis of features, modifications, and applications, In: Mathes SJ, Nahai F, eds. *Reconstructive Surgery: Principles, Anatomy, and Technique.* New York, NY: Churchill Livingstone, 1997.

Uses

Primary: Description

Secondary: Treatment, Research

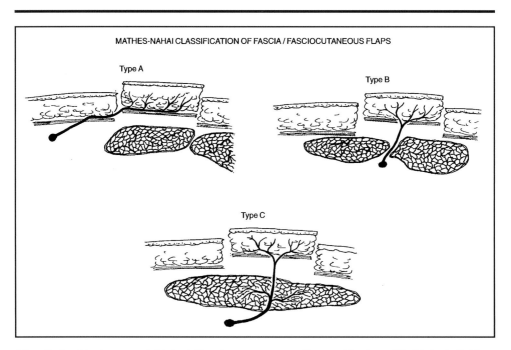

Fig 7–1. Mathes and Nahai fasciocutaneous flaps. Mathes SJ, Nahai F, Flap selection: analysis of features, modifications, and applications. In: Mathes SJ and Nahai F, eds, *Reconstructive Surgery: Principles, Anatomy, and Technique.* New York, NY: Churchill Livingstone; 1997. Copyright by Elsevier. Reprinted with permission.

Limited/none: Etiology, Prognosis, Diagnosis

Comments

Dr. Paul Oxley

Similar in its application as Cormack and Lamberty's, this system is a basic classification of local and free fasciocutaneous flaps. Each area of the skin gets its blood supply from a specific source, areas known as angiosomes.

The above system looks at how the blood gets from a major vessel to the skin, whether directly or via a septum or muscle. As perforator flaps are becoming more and more common, this classification is getting more attention, and has been further subdivided.

Essentially, it defines the blood supply of flaps and therefore their usefulness in certain reconstructive situations. The system is applied preoperatively to determine how a flap is raised and where it might be useful. It is slightly easier to use than Cormack and Lamberty's scheme as it is a better defined system.

Dr. Fu-Chan Wei and Dr. Perry Liu

This is an outdated classification system that was devised prior to the advent of the perforator flap concept. It limits the current understanding and advancement of free-flap surgery. The evolution of free cutaneous flaps have progressed from direct or septocutaneous vessel flaps → myocutaneous flaps → perforator flaps → free-style free flaps.

Only those that take an intramuscular course can be named as perforator. I prefer to classify skin vessels as direct vessels, septocutaneous vessels, and myocutaneous perforators. The distinction between septocutaneous vessels and myocutaneous perforators is whether the vascular pedicle takes an intramuscular course and requiring intramuscular pedicle dissection during flap harvest.

Muscle Flaps (Mathes and Nahai)

What It Classifies

Blood flow into muscles.

AKA

Mathes-Nahai classification of muscle or musculocutaneous flaps

System

I: Single dominant vessel (eg, gastrocnemius, tensor fascia lata)

II: Single dominant vessel with minor vessel contribution (eg, trapezius, gracilis)

III: Two dominant vessels (eg, rectus abdominus, gluteus maximus)

IV: Multiple segmental perforators (eg serratus). No use as free flaps.

V: One dominant and multiple segmentals capable of keeping muscle perfused (eg, pectoralis major, latissimus dorsi)

See Figure 7-2.

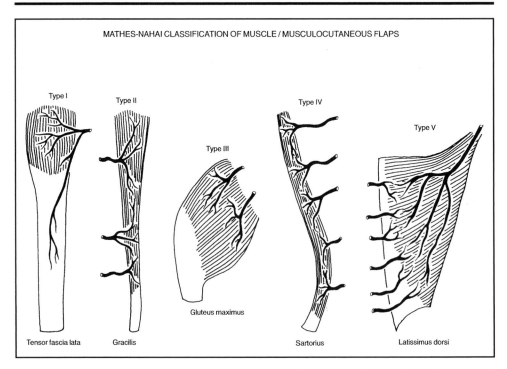

Fig 7–2. Mathes and Nahai muscle flaps. Mathes SJ, Nahai F. Classification of the vascular anatomy of muscles: experimental and clinical correlation. *Plast Reconstr Surg.* 1981;67:177. Copyright by Elsevier. Reprinted with permission.

References

Ger R. *Current Problems in Surgery.* Chicago, Ill: Year Book; 1972.

Mathes SJ, Nahai F. Classification of the vascular anatomy of muscles: experimental and clinical correlation. *Plast Reconstr Surg.* 1981;67:177.

Mathes SJ, Nahai F. Flap selection: analysis of features, modifications, and applications, In: Mathes SJ and Nahai F, eds. *Reconstructive Surgery: Principles, Anatomy, and Technique.* New York, NY: Churchill Livingstone, 1997.

Uses

Primary: Description

Secondary: Treatment, Research

Limited/none: Etiology, Prognosis, Diagnosis

Comments

Dr. Paul Oxley

This classification system is the most widely used for defining local and free muscle flaps. It describes the type of blood supply a muscle receives, whether from single or multiple vessels and from dominant, codominant, or minor vessels. Understanding the different blood supply of muscles helps determine which ones can reliably be used for free tissue transfer or as local pedicle flaps.

All major muscles in the body have been described using this classification. This information, along with the potential functional loss of taking that muscle, helps determine which muscles can be used in reconstruction.

This is a descriptive classification only and its use is in directing treatment of damaged areas. Exact options depend on the location and size of a defect, patient factors such as vascular disease or diabetes, and the willingness to accept donor site morbidity.

Dr. Martin Jugenburg and Dr. Andrea Pusic

Muscle flaps have traditionally been used because of their excellent vascularity to cover difficult wounds (eg, latissimus dorsi, rectus abdominis), or as carriers of the overlying fasciocutaneous component (eg, latissimus dorsi and TRAM in breast reconstruction). Muscle flaps were initially described by Ger, and subsequently classified based on their vascular supply by Mathes and Nahai.

This classification describes the type of blood supply a muscle receives, whether from single or multiple vessels and from dominant, codominant, or minor vessels. Understanding the different blood supply of muscles helps determine which ones can reliably be used in free tissue transfers and pedicle flaps. Each muscle in the body has been described using this classification. This information, along with the potential functional loss of taking that muscle helps determine which muscles can be used in reconstruction.

Type I muscles have a single dominant vessel and thus inclusion of this vessel in the flap ensures excellent perfusion to the flap. Type II flaps such as gracilis can be elevated on the dominant vessel, and the segment dependent on the minor vessel contribution can usually be safely included assuming it is only one angiosome away from the dominant vessel-supplied area. Type III muscles have two dominant vessels. In the case of rectus abdominis, for example, the blood supply is sufficient to maintain the entire muscle, but overlying fasciocutaneous segment is less reliable. Pedicled TRAM flaps are based on the superior epigastric vessels, whereas the adipocutaneous part of the TRAM flap is primarily supplied by the inferior epigastric vessels. Therefore, pedicle TRAM flaps are more prone to fat necrosis (as a result of poorer blood supply) than free TRAM flaps where the inferior epigastric vessel is the inflow vessel into the flap. Type IV flaps have segmental perforators and should not be used as flaps. Sternocleidomastoid muscle is an example of such a flap. It has been described in the past for use in H/N reconstruction, but due to its unreliability it is rarely used. Type V flaps are pectoralis major and latissimus dorsi. These flaps can be raised either on the dominant blood supply or on the segmental blood supply (however, one must ensure that as many as possible of these segmental perforators are preserved) (Fig 7–3).

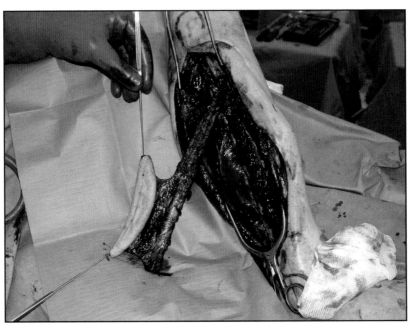

A

Fig 7–3. Fibula flap for reconstruction of mandible **A.** Harvest
continues

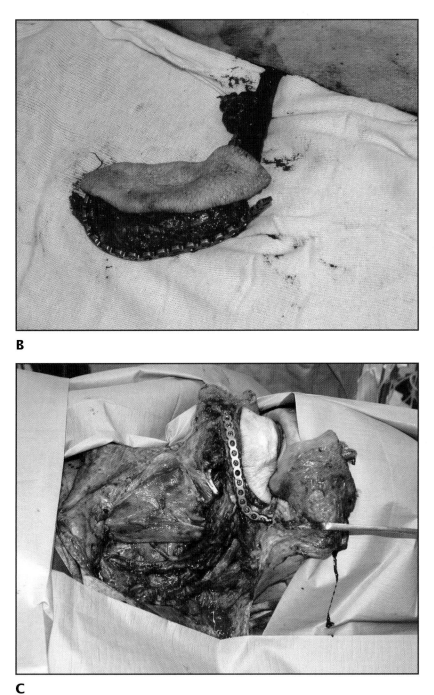

B

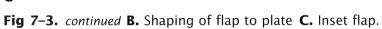

C

Fig 7–3. *continued* **B.** Shaping of flap to plate **C.** Inset flap.

Maxillectomy and Midfacial Defect Reconstruction

What It Classifies

The extent of the defect and possible options for reconstruction of maxillectomy and midfacial defects.

System

Type I: Limited maxillectomy

Resection of one or two walls of the maxilla excluding palate.

Usually anterior wall and either medial wall or orbital floor

Type II: Subtotal maxillectomy

Resection of maxillary arch, palate, anterior and lateral walls

Preservation of orbital floor

Type III: Total Maxillectomy

Resection of all 6 walls of maxilla

IIIa: Orbital contents preserved

IIIb: Orbital contents exenterated

Type IV: Orbitomaxillectomy

Exenteration of orbit and resection of upper 5 walls of maxilla

Preservation of palate

References

Cordeiro PG, Santamaria E. A classification system and algorithm for reconstruction of maxillectomy and midfacial defects. *Plast Reconstr Surg.* 2000;105(7):2331–2346.

Brown JS, Rogers SN, McNally DN, et al. A modified classification for the maxillectomy defect. *Head Neck.* 2000;22:17–26.

Futran ND, Alsarraf R. Microvascular free-flap reconstruction in the head and neck. *JAMA.* 2000;284:1761–1763.

Futran ND, Mendez E. Developments in reconstruction of midface and maxilla. *Lancet Oncol.* 2006;7:249–258.

Wells MD, Luce EA. Reconstruction of midfacial defects after surgical resection of malignancies. *Clin Plast Surg.* 1995;22:79–89.

Uses

Primary: Description, Treatment, Research

Secondary: Diagnosis, Prognosis

Limited/none: Etiology

Comments

Dr. Paul Oxley

The reconstructive challenges following partial or complete resection of the midface can be daunting. Many structures need to be addressed, including bone and soft tissue defects. The authors of this study looked at the effects of the loss of various structures and the most effective way of planning reconstruction.

This system critically breaks down the potential defects into four groups, each with specific issues. The key point is the extent of maxilla remaining after resection. The paper also suggests options for reconstruction based on an algorithm. Essentially, this focuses first on bone, then soft tissue (including skin, palate and cheek lining), and finally specialized structures (eg, eyelids). Further details of the proposed algorithm are found in the original paper.

This classification is an excellent tool for assessing the reconstructive challenges of midfacial resection. It clearly defines the levels of severity and leaves little open for interpretation. Using this system, one is able to easily describe the defect as well as apply that information toward treatment options. It is also useful as a research tool for similar reasons.

Dr. Colleen McCarthy

The broad category of maxillectomy represents a wide spectrum of diverse defects. The approach to reconstruction of midfacial defects is further complicated due to the disparate shapes and sizes of tumors affecting the maxilla, the complex three-dimensional anatomy, and the contiguous relationship of the maxilla to the surrounding structures.

Attesting to both the variety and complexity of midfacial defects, numerous different classification systems exist (by Brown, Wells, Futran). Although the majority of these aforementioned schemas provide accurate—and in some cases extremely detailed—descriptions of post-ablative defects of the midface, many do not provide clear direction regarding treatment options. In addition, many of these schemas do not include important structures such as the orbit and/or zygoma.

This current classification system by Cordeiro et al is principally based on the extent of resection of the maxillary bone. Defects of the midface are primarily categorized according to which walls of the maxilla are resected. Further subclassification is then made based on the assessment of the associated soft-tissue, skin, palatal, cheek, and mucosal deficits. Conceptually, Cordeiro et al describe the

maxilla as a geometric structure with six walls - a hexahedron. The roof of the box is the floor of the orbit; the floor forms the anterior hard palate and alveolar ridge. The medial wall forms the lateral wall of the nasal cavity and is a part of the lacrimal system. The maxillary sinus, the largest of the paranasal sinuses, is contained within the central portion of the maxilla. Overlying the posterior pterygoid region of the maxilla is the cranial base.

For type I defects, the author prefers the radial forearm fasciocutaneous flap. If critical segments of bone are missing, such as the orbital rim or the anterior floor of the orbit, nonvascularized bone grafts can provide the needed support. For type II defects, the osteocutaneous "sandwich" forearm flap is used. The rectus abdominis free flap used in combination with nonvascularized bone grafts is preferred for type IIIA defects; the rectus abdominis free flap is similarly preferred for type IIIB defects. Finally, the rectus abdmoninis free flap provides adequate tissue requirements and an adequate pedicle length for type IV defects.

In summary, the system succinctly groups a wide array of possible composite tissue defects and can easily be used to facilitate clinical decision-making by outlining preferred reconstructive options and their common functional and aesthetic sequelae. This comprehensive approach has simplified the ability to understand, describe, and communicate the nature of these often complex reconstructive problems.

Dr. Fu-Chan Wei and
Dr. Perry Liu

This is the most common and popular system for classifying maxillary and midfacial defects. However, this classification system fails to take into account the re-section and reconstruction of the upper dentures in type I defects. Simple soft tissue reconstruction of maxillary defects involving the upper dentures is insufficient. These defects require alveolar bone replacement for placement of dental implants. In Taiwan, most of our patients fall into the type I or type II categories. Type I and type II defects are usually due to oral cavity tumors. Type III and IV defects are usually caused by osteosarcomas, orbital, and brain tumors.

Most of the reconstructive options detailed by Cordeiro involve upper trunk flaps. We prefer to use lower trunk options such as the ALT and fibular flaps for these reconstructions. For example, in Figure 5 of his paper, we would use the ALT flap for the 1st, 3rd, and 4th case scenarios. The fibular flap would be used for the 2nd scenario. In our practice, the ALT has supplanted both the rectus abdominus and radial forearm flaps. The fibula is the ideal choice when bony reconstruction is necessary. Using lower body/trunk flaps allow us to utilize two teams for the surgery and decrease operative time.

Periorbital Surgical Zones

What It Classifies

Surgical zones around the orbits including eyelids and periorbital skin.

System

Zone I: On the upper eyelid

Zone II: On the lower eyelid

Zone III: On the medial canthal region

Zone IV: On the lateral canthal region

Zone V: Outside but contiguous with zones I to IV

See Figure 7-4.

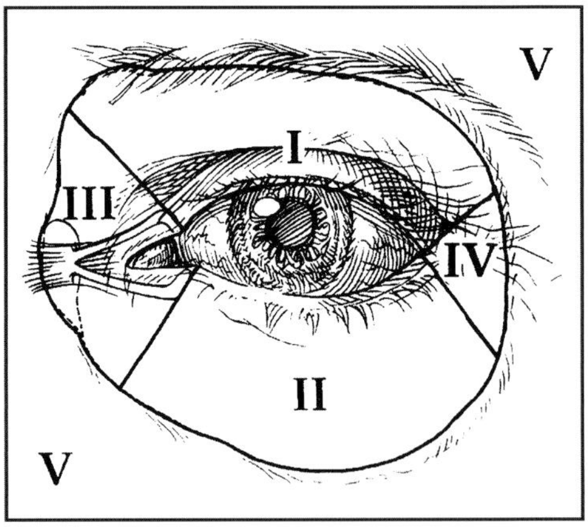

Fig 7–4. Periorbital surgical zones. Glat PM, Longaker MT, Jelks EB, et al. Periorbital melanocytic lesions: excision and reconstruction in 40 patients. *Plast Reconstr Surg.* 1998;102(1): 19–27. Copyright 1998 by Lippincott, Williams & Wilkins. Reprinted with permission.

References

Glat PM, Longaker MT, Jelks EB, et al. Periorbital melanocytic lesions: excision and reconstruction in 40 patients. *Plast Reconstr Surg.* 1998;102(1):19–27.

Spinelli HM, Jelks GW. Periocular reconstruction: a systematic approach. *Plast Reconstr Surg.* 1993;91:1017.

Uses

Primary: Description, Research

Secondary: Treatment

Limited/none: Diagnosis, Prognosis, Etiology

Comments

Dr. Paul Oxley

The management of periorbital tumours or post-traumatic defects can be challenging. There are several options for reconstructing parts or all of an affected area. This system accepts that each zone is treated differently. The authors first provided a schema for dividing these tissues into zones (1993) and then in the later paper (1998) applied that system to help describe reconstructive options used in their study.

The system is a simple one and easy to apply. Although it does not have any modifiers for things such as complete or incomplete, or which part of a zone is affected in the case of Zones I or II, it does help to structure the approach to reconstruction. It also assists in record keeping for the purpose of research into effective means of periorbital reconstruction.

Venous Flaps (Thatte and Thatte)

What It Classifies

Flaps that are based on a venous rather than an arterial pedicle.

System

Type 1: Supplied by a single venous pedicle

Type 2: Venous flow-through flaps. Flap based on a single vein that carries blood in and out of the flap

Type 3: Arterialized venous flaps

Reference

Thatte MR, Thatte RL. Venous flaps. *Plast Reconstr Surg.* 1993;91(4):747–751.

Uses

Primary: Research, Description

Secondary: Treatment

Limited/none: Diagnosis, Prognosis, Etiology

Comments

Dr. Paul Oxley

Flaps, whether pedicled or free, are defined by the type of blood supply that nourishes them. In arterial flaps, this is determined by the manner in which a vessel reaches the fasciocutaneous tissue or the dominance of a given blood vessel to the muscle it feeds. Venous flaps are rarely used in most centers, as arterial flaps are preferred in most cases. This is likely due to the familiarity with these flaps and the robust blood supply provided by arteries.

Nevertheless, venous flaps should be familiar to the reconstructive surgeon as they may be the best option in some circumstances.

This classification system is, like venous flaps themselves, seldom used. The classification system describes the flow characteristics of the different types of venous flaps. Due to the relative underuse of these flaps when compared to arterial flaps, this classification is useful in clarifying which type of flap was utilized in a given situation and standardizing research in this area.

Classification of V-Y Plasty

What It Classifies

V-Y Plasty and its analogues.

System

See Table 7–3 and Figure 7–5.

Reference

Suzuki S, Matsuda K, Nishimura Y. Proposal for a new comprehensive classification of V-Y plasty and its analogues: the pros and cons of inverted versus ordinary Burow's triangle excision. *Plast Reconstr Surg.* 1996;98(6):1016–1022.

Uses

Primary: Treatment

Secondary: Description

Limited/none: Etiology, Diagnosis, Research, Prognosis

Comments

Dr. Paul Oxley

The movement of soft tissue for wound coverage or scar release can be complex. Suzuki et al attempt here to simplify the classification of local soft tissue advancement using one or more V-Y flaps with or without the removal of true or inverted Burow's triangles. Burow's triangles are designed to help facilitate the advancement of the V-flap and reduce dog-ear formation.

This system can be easily applied not only to soft tissue coverage but also in scar tissue release. In the latter it is useful

Table 7–3. V-Y Plasty

V-Y
▪ Burrow's triangles often applied as advocated by Limberg.
▪ 5-Z plasty
Double V-Y
▪ Inverted Burrow's triangles can also be used
– Resembles Koyama and Fukimori's V-W plasty
▪ 7-Z plasty
▪ Division of a wide V-flap into two V-flaps
i. Two Y-W flap described by Borges commenting on V-W flap
ii. V-M plasty = double V-Y with paired inverted Burrow's (Alexander)

Source: From "Proposal for a new comprehensive classification of V-Y plasty and its analogues: the pros and cons of inverted versus ordinary Burow's triangle excision," Suzuki S, Matsuda K, Nishimura Y, *Plast Reconstr Surg.* 1996;98(6), pp. 1016–1022. Copyright 1996 by Lippincott, Williams & Wilkins. Reprinted with permission.

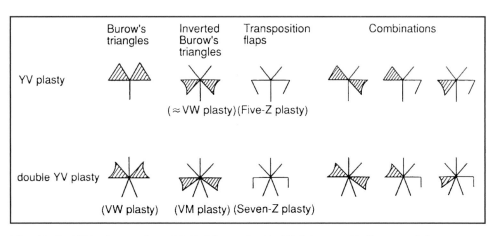

Fig 7–5. V-Y plasty. Suzuki S, Matsuda K, Nishimura Y. Proposal for a new comprehensive classification of V-Y plasty and its analogues: the pros and cons of inverted versus ordinary Burow's triangle excision. *Plast Reconstr Surg.* 1996;98(6):1016–1022. Copyright 1996 by Lippincott, Williams & Wilkins. Reprinted with permission.

in reminding the surgeon of options to best incorporate healthy skin while maximizing clinical outcome.

Dr. Adrian Lee

A classification is for communications. When broadly accepted, it allows us to accurately categorize and convey a topic to others in a succinct manner. For a classification to be broadly accepted, it must be inclusive of all variables, yet simple for recall. It should efficiently stratify a topic in increasing complexity and, in the case of medicine, correspondingly guide treatment.

This classification of V-Y plasties attempts to organize this particular local flap from simple to complex. Its focus is on the geometry and preoperative planning as opposed to when one should be used over another. As the authors have pointed out, increasing number of simultaneous V-Y flaps lead to greater release of a contracture, but at the expense of increasing risk of vascular compromise due to ever smaller flaps. This contradiction leaves us in a state of limbo as to what to do. The classification seems to suggest that the greater the contracture, the greater the number of V-Y flaps that have to be done, yet clinically, this may be ill-advised. Consequently, the classification has not effectively helped us in a treatment plan. Furthermore, this classification is cumbersome and difficult to recall without diagrams, which would undermine general acceptance and usage. In the end, although studying and understanding the classification is a good mental exercise in geometry, its clinical value is questionable, and is therefore not very useful.

Chapter 8

TRAUMA

Burn Alopecia

What It Classifies

Extent of alopecia secondary to a burn and its ability to be treated by tissue expansion.

System

See Table 8-1.

Reference

McCauley RL. Correction of burn alopecia. In: Herndon DN, ed. *Total Burn Care*. 2nd ed. Philadelphia, Pa: W.B. Saunders; 2002: 690-694.

Uses

Primary: Description, Treatment

Secondary: Research, Diagnosis, Prognosis

Limited/none: Etiology

Comments

Dr. Paul Oxley

This classification is used to direct the treatment of alopecia following thermal

Table 8-1. Burn Alopecia

Type	Segments
I	Single alopecia segment amenable to tissue expansion
	Ia Single segment <25% of hair bearing scalp
	Ib Single segment 25–50%
	Ic Single segment 50–75%
	Id Single segment >75%
II	Multiple areas amenable to tissue expansion
III	Patchy burn alopecia not amenable to tissue expansion
IV	Total alopecia

Source: From "Correction of burn alopecia," McCauley RL. In: Herndon DN, ed, *Total Burn Care*, 2nd ed., Philadelphia, Pa: W.B. Saunders; 2002:690–694. Copyright 2002 by Elsevier. Reprinted with permission.

injury, largely with the use of tissue expanders. It classifies the size of the defect first and then from that offers suggestions for the user of tissue expanders required for appropriate defects. Whether the area is amenable to tissue expansion usually refers to the presence of an area of hair baring skin in a location useful for reconstruction and large enough to place a tissue expander under. Obviously, whether the alopecia has bare skin on all sides versus one or two makes a difference with respect to the ability to cover the area with expanded skin.

The treatment of burn alopecia tends to be largely surgeon dependent. Where one surgeon might use a single expander another may use two. The location of the alopecia can affect the best options for treatment as the anterior scalp is treated differently from the posterior scalp. Rotation flaps are often used instead of tissue expansion to move hair to more aesthetic locations (eg, frontal hairline).

The system has some use in research by giving specific numbers for the defects, however narrowing down to an exact percentage can be difficult with a rounded surface like the scalp. The biggest problem with this classification is its lack of site specificity.

Dr. E. E. Tredget

This classification is authored by Dr. Robert McCauley who has very broad experience in the management of alopecia, particularly in the pediatric burn population. This classification is generally accepted by leaders in the burn field and reasonably describes the type of defect and the application of soft tissue expansion for its surgical correction.

Burn Depth

What It Classifies

Depth of burn with respect to histologic depth, or also known as degree of burn.

System

1st Degree: Burn extends no deeper than epidermis. Red, painful, nonblistered appearance. Dry, minimal edema. Usually heals in 7 to 10 days with no scarring.

2nd Degree: Burn extends in to dermis. Dermal appendages maintained which allows for self-healing. Epidermal sloughing. Blisters present. Usually red in appearance, painful, and moist. Usually heals in 7 to 14 days with minimal scarring. Deeper burns may require surgery to prevent severe scarring.

3rd Degree: Burn extends through dermis. All dermal appendages lost. Blisters may be present. Insensate, nonexpandable skin. Variable color—red, black, white, brown, gray—usually hard leathery or woody to palpation. Requires secondary intention or surgery to heal.

4th Degree: Burn extends into subcutaneous soft tissue other than fat (eg, muscle, bone, nerve). Appearance and pain level similar to 3rd degree.

Reference

Press B, Thermal, electrical, and chemical injuries In: Aston SJ, Beasley RW, Thorne CHM, eds. *Grabb and Smith's Plastic Surgery*. 5th ed. Philadelphia Pa: Lippincott-Raven Publishers; 1997:161.

Uses

Primary: Description, Diagnosis,

Secondary: Prognosis, Treatment, Research

Limited/none: Etiology

Comments

Dr. Paul Oxley

Depth is the gold standard for description of cutaneous thermal injury: it is almost universally understood. Early burn management is based on the extent and depth of the burn in most cases. Accurate early determination of burn depth is difficult in some cases, especially differentiating between deep second and third degree burns. Some specific types of burns such as oil burns are more difficult to predict than others. In some instances, the wound is observed over 1 to 2 weeks to determine the exact depth of injury.

Early treatment and prognosis is largely related to burn depth and extent of total body surface area burned. Other factors play important roles in the prediction of outcome including the location of the burn, patient age, comorbid injury or illness, and the time to and adequacy of initial treatment. Some characteristics specific to burns, such as smoke inhalation and source of burn injury (eg, electrical burn), will also have an important role in determining treatment and prognosis.

Some centers use the term "partial thickness burn" in place of second degree, and divide those into superficial or deep. Under this system, "full thickness" replaces the term "third degree." This change refers to the histologic depth more specifically and descriptively than the degree classification. By subdividing the second degree burns into two categories it recognizes the different management of the burns and the possibility of worse scarring following deeper burns (Fig 8-1).

Dr. Charles Snelling

What has been called second degree burns is normally recognized as having two subgroups. These are: superficial second degree, generally healing in 14 days with minimal or no scarring; and deep second degree, usually healing after 14 to 21 days with likely significant scarring.

Sometimes second degree is referred to as partial thickness with superficial partial thickness and deep partial thickness as the subgroups, whereas third degree is full thickness. Sometimes second degree is subdivide into superficial dermal and dermal corresponding with the above mentioned healing times. I think that recognition of the subclassification within second degree, by one or more terms, is crucial.

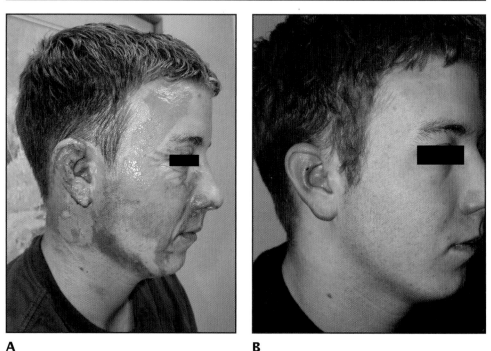

A   **B**

Fig 8–1. A. Superficial second degree facial burn following firework explosion. **B.** Healed spontaneously after 10 days.

Dr. E. E. Tredget

This system is nicely outlined in the materials provided and has an accompanying reference which is reasonable but somewhat outdated and many more complete texts on the subject exist. However, the classification of burn depth is time-honored and practical in terms of the injury to skin and what is found histologically. Although this system cannot be replaced, many burn centers and physicians employ a practical approach toward the classification of depth of burn injury to partial thickness and full thickness injuries which categorizes patients as to whether they would benefit from split thickness skin graft or be allowed to heal their wounds spontaneously. Partial thickness are subdivided into superficial and deep, and although this approach is complicated by the difficulty in diagnosing intermediate depth dermal injury, the advent of scanning laser Doppler burn depth assessment equipment has begun to objectify and more accurately diagnose these injuries. This is important in that this alternative classification of burn depth aims to recognize second degree burn injuries that in the deeper wounds will often go on to develop significant amounts of hypertrophic scarring which could be avoided by intervening with a skin graft. A series of new scanning laser Dopplers and infrared technology is being applied for more accurate diagnosis of the depth of partial thickness injuries which will make this more objective and more important in the future. One of many references to these technologies which will aid in the refinement of classification of burn depth includes *Burns*, 2006;32:550-553, by Lahei entitled "Laser Doppler Imaging of Pediatric Burn Wound Outcome Can Be Predicted Independent of Clinical Examination."

In addition, burn depth together with total body surface area involved is used to prognosticate the severity of injury, to predict fluid requirements for fluid resuscitation during the early burn shock phase of injury, and for prognostication for survival dependent on severity of injury. It is often poorly appreciated that the depth of burn injury is a critical factor in predicting severity of injury. Traditionally, many formulas fail to differentiate depth of injury and appreciate its importance. For example, for a second degree superficial scald burn, which is superficial involving 95% of the total body surface area involves a much smaller mass of dead and injured tissue than a deep, full thickness burn injury involving 80% of the total body surface area. The latter injury is not considered differently by any of the many fluid resuscitation formulas used to calculate resuscitation requirements but the practical reality is that they are considerably different in terms of the actual amounts of fluids that will be required and substantially different in predicting outcome and survival after burn injury. Thus, many publications are emerging to substantiate it is the amount of full-thickness burn injury that is very much more important in determining the severity of injury.

Burn Type

What It Classifies

The cause of a burn.

System

1. Flame: Burn due to direct contact with flame
2. Scald: Burn due to direct contact with hot fluid (water, oil, tar)
3. Radiation: Burn due to exposure to radiation source such as nuclear fuel or the sun
4. Contact: Burn due to contact with a hot structure (eg, stove element)
5. Electrical: Burn due to exposure to electrical current either by direct contact or by arcing of current into body. Includes lightning
6. Chemical: Burn due to contact with either acid or alkali substance

Reference

Press B. Thermal, electrical, and chemical injuries. In: Aston SJ, Beasley RW, Thorne CHM, eds. *Grabb and Smith's Plastic Surgery.* 5th ed. Philadelphia, Pa: Lippincott-Raven Publishers; 1997:161.

Uses

Primary: Etiology, Treatment,

Secondary: Description, Diagnosis, Research

Limited/none: Prognosis

Comments

Dr. Paul Oxley

This is a simple way of looking at the cause of burn, each with a slightly different approach to the immediate management. It is vital in the early management of a burn to know the cause of the injury, not just for the sake of the patient but also for those helping in the case of chemical burns.

Defining the type of burn injury gives the referring and receiving physicians a simple way to describe the cause of the injury, and to direct best methods of care. Some types of injury have other inherent concerns, such as inhalation injury in the cases of flame burns.

Prognosis depends on multiple factors, including the burn type, the location and total body surface area burned, and the presence of other injuries. The type of injury and the treatment given for it are key factors.

Dr. Charles Snelling

This classification deals with etiology and I think that there are more headings that should be included. I would first clarify that electrical burns have three separate entities with a fourth being a combination of the other three. These would be flash, contact, and flame burns with electrical energy as the primary source. Flash is due to heat produced by the electrical current without contact to the patient. Contact refers to the direct arcing of electricity through the patient.

I feel it is important to further separate lightning from other electrical burns. Lastly, the flame burn would be as a result of clothing catching fire due to electrical current.

Other categories that I would include would be hot oil burns which generally have a very high temperature and need to be treated differently from basic scald burns. The next would be tar burns with an even higher temperature still and more difficult treatment than oil or scald burns. I would add a category for sunburns which I believe are different from radiation burns, though some sources consider the sunburn a type of radiation burn. Lastly, I would add friction burns as a final etiologic type.

The reason for differentiating these is that there are specific initial emergency treatments for some of these which might not be obvious if they are contained in a larger, nonspecific group.

Dr. E.E. Tredget

As discussed by Dr. Oxley above, the mechanism or pathophysiology which accounts for the thermal injury to the skin is important for many aspects of treatment, management, and understanding the nature of injury. The types of injury is reasonable, complete, and classically found in most standard texts because it is practical, simple, and descriptive. In reality, the difficulty lies in the management and understanding the subtypes and range of severity that exist in electrical injury, specific chemical injuries, and radiation injury where the range of severity and the pathophysiology can be broadly different depending on the severity of injury.

Vancouver Burn Scar Score

What It Classifies

The extent of scarring following a burn injury and subsequent healing.

AKA

Vancouver Scar Scale, Burn Scar Score

System

See Table 8–2.

Reference

Sullivan T, Smith J, Kermode J, McIver E, Coutemanche DJ. Rating the burn scar. *J Burn Care Rehab*. 1990;11:256–260.

Uses

Primary: Diagnosis, Description, Research

Secondary: Treatment, Prognosis

Limited/none: Etiology

Comments

Dr. Paul Oxley

Most classification systems for trauma focus on the immediate problem from the injury, for example, the depth of burn or the type of fracture. Instead, this classification addresses the healing process that follows injury. The severity of scars in the burn patient has a significant impact on the patient's quality of life after the event. It is generally difficult to rate one scar versus another without very objective criteria.

Developed at the BC Firefighter's Burn Unit in Vancouver, Canada, this burn scar classification, or more precisely a scoring system, was designed to help objectively rate a scar for the purpose of standardizing treatment and research. Each characteristic of the scar is given a number

Table 8–2. Vancouver Burn Scar Score

Pigmentation	Vascularity	Pliability	Height	Score
Normal	Normal	Normal	Normal	0
Hypopigmentation	Pink	Supple	Raised <2 mm	1
Hyperpigmentation	Red	Yielding	Raised 2–5 mm	2
	Purple	Firm	Raised >5 mm	3
		Banding		4
		Contracture		5

Source: From "Rating the burn scar," Sullivan T, Smith J, Kermode J, McIver E, Coutemanche DJ. *J Burn Care Rehab*. 1990;11:256–260. Copyright 1990 by Lippincott, Williams & Wilkins. Reprinted with permission.

value, with those values added and the higher the score, the worse the scar.

The treatment and prognosis will depend on the score, but will also be influenced by factors such as scar location, size, and comorbid conditions (Fig 8–2).

Dr. Doug Courtemanche

The value of the Burn Scar Score is in the long-term evaluation of scars in the burn survivor. Scoring scars over time allows for an objective assessment of scar maturation and a focus on scars that need more attention (operative or nonoperative intervention).

This paper is frequently cited and the score scale has been modified by other authors. It has been extended to non-burn scars and the scar symptoms have been included, scored, and reported. All of these small changes have increased our understanding of the impact of scars on burn survivors and other patients (eg, cancer survivors).

Use of this system for evaluating scars of selected patients, or groups of patients, for care or research will continue. The system is based on the practical application of an understanding of wound healing and scar maturation.

Dr Charles Snelling

The key element of this sytem is that the evaluation of a scar can be repeated to track the progress of the scar since time of creation and to track the effectiveness of specific scar treatment.

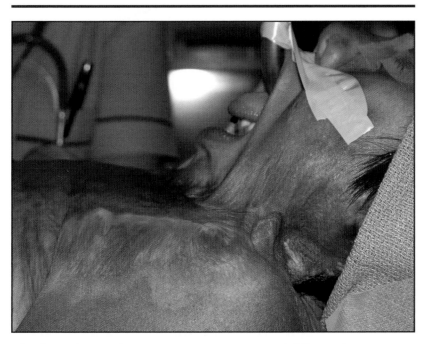

Fig 8–2. Severe burn scar contracture in child's neck.

Facial Blunt Trauma Soft-Tissue Damage

What It Classifies

Blunt trauma induced soft tissue injury of the face.

AKA

"MCFONTZL," pronounced MACFONS-EL

System

See Table 8-3 and Figure 8-3.
   Severity score then calculated for each laceration using the numbers at T, E, R, I, and S:

   T + E + R + I + S = severity score

Grading the score:

   MCFONTZL Class I:
   Severity score 1 to 5

   MCFONTZL Class II:
   Severity score 6 to 10

   MCFONTZL Class III:
   Severity score 11 to 15

   MCFONTZL Class IV:
   Severity score greater than 15

Repeated for each laceration

Reference

Lee RH, Gamble WB, Robertson B, Manson PN. The MCFONTZL classification system for soft-tissue injuries to the face. *Plast Reconstr Surg*. 1999;103(4):1150–1157.

Uses

Primary: Description, Diagnosis

Secondary: Research, Treatment

Limited/none: Etiology, Prognosis

Comments

Dr. Paul Oxley

Classifying soft tissue injuries is very difficult (Fig 8-4) and few systems exist that have been readily accepted and applied. The problem lies in the huge variability that can be encountered in any given injury and trying to put a numeric value on the injury. Most classifications focus on deficits or injury to underlying tissue.

   Lee et al propose a classification that at first seems very confusing, though when one takes the time to go through the system, it is actually very easy to apply. Start by drawing a schematic face and place an 8-point asterisk at the site of each laceration. One then fills in the information as described above. Once each value is determined the severity score is quickly calculated.

   This system helps give a better record in a simple fashion than can be created by drawing or trying to verbally describe each laceration. It can be used by people unfamiliar with CPT codes, simply by ignoring the last point on the asterisk. Its biggest limitation is how to best describe extensive lacerations crossing many zones. Its cumbersome appearance makes it less likely to be adapted into practice by some.

Table 8–3. MCFONTZL

Location of Injury

  M: Maxilla

  C: Chin

  F: Forehead

  O: Orbit

  N: Nose

  T: Temple

  Z: Zygoma

  L: Lip (excluding intraoral lacerations)

Extent/Type of Laceration

  A: Area
- Location of index laceration as denoted by the MCFONTZL unit.
- Index laceration is the dominant laceration with maximum, continuous skin interruption.
- If it extends into a different anatomic unit, it is assigned to the unit representing the zone of impact or maximum interuuption.

  S: Side
- Side of the unit: Right, Left, Center (forehead), Upper, and Lower

  T: Thickness
- Depth of penetration: Epidermis (E), Dermis (D), Subcutaneous fat (F), Muscle (M), Bone (B)
- Number values are given for scoring (E = 0, D = 1, F = 2, M = 3, B = 4)

  E: Extension
- Number of branches from index laceration greater than 1.0 cm long

  R: Relaxed skin tension line
- Is the vector of the index laceration along Langer's lines (0 = yes, 1 = no)

  I: Index laceration
- Length of the index laceration in centimeters

  S: Soft tissue defect
- Tissue loss from complete avulsion: 0 = none, 1 = 1 cm radius along long axis, 2 = 2 cm radius along long axis, etc.

  K: CPT coding
- based on depth and length of laceration

Each letter is notated along each ray of a modified asterisk symbol starting with *A* at twelve o'clock and rotating clockwise with each letter written at the end of each ray.

Source: From "The MCFONTZL classification system for soft-tissue injuries to the face," Lee RH, Gamble WB, Robertson B, Manson PN. *Plast Reconstr Surg.* 1999;103(4):1150–1157. Copyright 1999 by Lippincott, Williams & Wilkins. Reprinted with permission.

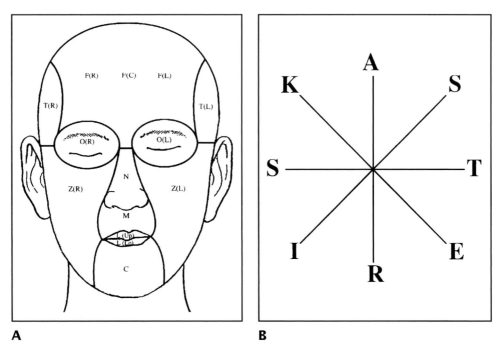

A

B

Fig 8–3. A. Regions of the face. **B.** Asterisk pattern. Lee RH, Gamble WB, Robertson B, Manson PN. The MCFONTZL classification system for soft-tissue injuries to the face. *Plast Reconstr Surg.* 1999;103(4):1150–1157. Copyright 1999 by Lippincott, Williams & Wilkins. Reprinted with permission.

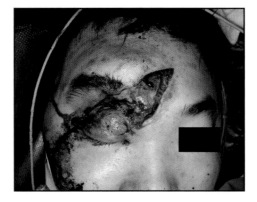

Fig 8–4. Severe periorbital laceration following contact with windshield. MCFONTZL Class IV (A = orbit, S = L, T = 4, E = O, R = 1, I = 11, S = 0, Total = 16).

Frontal Basilar Trauma

What It Classifies

Fractures to the frontal, orbit, and temporal bones as well as those also involving the ethmoid complex.

System

Type I (Central): Confined to the upper nasoethmoidal complex, central frontal bone, and medial third of the superior orbital rims with bilateral frontal sinus involvement.

Type II (Unilateral): Involves the entire supraorbital rim and the upper lateral orbital wall, extending into the squamosa of the temporal bone and ipsilateral frontal bone and unilateral frontal sinus fractures.

Type III (Bilateral): Involves fractures of the upper nasal ethmoidal complex, bilateral supraorbital and upper lateral orbital wall fractures, and bilateral frontal bone fractures and the entire frontal sinus.

Reference

Burstein F, Cohen S, Hudgins R, Boydston W. Frontal basilar trauma: classification and treatment. *Plast Reconstr Surg.* 1997; 99(5):1314-1321.

Uses

Primary: Description, Diagnosis, Treatment

Secondary: Research

Limited/none: Prognosis, Etiology

Comments

Dr. Paul Oxley

These fractures can be difficult to treat and may be overwhelming to the inexperienced surgeon. This classification was devised to facilitate the diagnosis and treatment of the injury by suggesting an algorithm for each fracture pattern. It was derived using CT images and categorizes fractures from a surgical correction point of view, grouping fractures to best plan operative repair. The classification can be used to plan elective orbital and cranial osteotomies that then can be employed for easier access to the fracture areas and facilitate repair.

Dr. Oleh Antonyshyn

A classification system is clinically useful when it guides the diagnosis or management of a clinical problem. The management of frontal basilar trauma must address the following:

1. restoration of normal contour to the forehead, glabella, and supraorbital rims
2. diagnosis and management of CSF rhinorrhea
3. specific management of injury to the frontal sinus
4. diagnosis and management of associated intraorbital injury
5. diagnosis and management of associated intracranial injury

The classification system proposed by Burstein et al does not adequately address all of these issues. This classification system is limited by the following:

1. It is a classification system that is primarily designed to address frontal basilar fractures in children and adolescents aged 18 months to 18 years of age with a mean age of 9.5 years. In this population of patients, the impact resistance of bone is higher, frontal sinuses are absent or not fully developed, and the incidence of associated orbital apex injuries is higher than one would see in an adult population.

   The patterns of skeletal injury and associated trauma are different in the adult population.

2. The classification focuses on describing three different anatomic patterns of frontal bone and base of skull injuries that can be addressed by three different types of frontal orbital osteotomy.

   The classification, however, is not comprehensive, and fails to identify the majority of adult patients with frontobasilar injuries who require teatment other than osteotomy.

Therefore, this classification system does not apply to an adult population,

and does not provide a guide to the comprehensive management of patients with such injuries.

Craniofrontal fractures are best classified according to:

1. Anatomic location
   a. central (involving the frontal sinus)
   b. lateral (not involving the frontal sinus)

The best reference that describes the differing implications of a lateral as opposed to a central frontal injury is described in an article by Gruss JS, Pollock RA, Phillips JH, and Antonyshyn O. "Combined Injuries of the Cranium and Face." *British Journal of Plastic Surgery.* 1989;42(4):385–398.

2. Extent of frontal sinus involvement
   a. anterior wall
   b. posterior wall
   c. floor

The best reference that summarizes the classification of frontal sinus fractures and implications of treatment is the following: Rohrich RJ, Hollier LH, "Management of Frontal Sinus Fractures. Changing Concepts." *Clinics of Plastic Surgery.* 1992;19(1):219–232.

Glasgow Coma Scale

What It Classifies

The conscious state of a patient.

System

See Table 8–4.

Table 8–4. Glasgow Coma Scale

Action by Patient	Score
Eyes Opening	
Spontaneously	4
To Speech	3
To Pain	2
None	1
Best Verbal Response	
Oriented	5
Confused	4
Inappropriate	3
Incomprehensible	2
None	1
Best Motor Response	
Obeys commands	6
Localizes to pain	5
Withdraws from pain	4
Flexion to pain	3
Extension to pain	2
None	1

Source: From "Facial fractures," Manson PN, In: Aston SJ, Beasley RW, Thorne CHM, eds, *Grabb and Smith's Plastic Surgery*, 5th ed. Philadelphia, Pa: Lippincott-Raven Publishers;1997: 383. Copyright 1997 by Lippincott, Williams & Wilkins. Reprinted with permission.

References

Manson PN. Facial fractures. In: Aston SJ, Beasley RW, Thorne CHM, eds. *Grabb and Smith's Plastic Surgery*. 5th ed. Philadelphia, Pa: Lippincott-Raven Publishers; 1997:383.

Teasdale G, Jennett B. Assessment of coma and impaired consciousness. A practical scale. *Lancet*. 1974;2(7872):81–84.

Uses

Primary: Diagnosis, Description

Secondary: Research, Treatment, Prognosis

Limited/none: Etiology

Comments

Dr. Paul Oxley

The Glasgow Coma Scale (GCS) is the universally accepted way of describing the conscious state of a patient. It is one of the most commonly quoted classifications for trauma patients of all types. With this information a clinician is able to monitor the clinical status accurately and quickly. It is a very reliable and reproducible test. A patient receives a score out of 15. The GCS, along with initial causative diagnosis (eg, trauma, brain tumour), and patient comorbidities, allows experienced clinicians to determine prognosis. Some basic "rules" apply clinically with respect to the GCS. For example: "GCS of 8—intubate," though each clinical situation needs to be considered individually.

Comment should be made regarding the patient's clinical condition if appropriate. For example, some people will place a T next to a score if the patient is intubated (eg, 9T) as speech assessment is no longer possible. Also, severe facial injuries may prevent the ability to either talk normally or open ones eyes due to swelling.

Scores are given based on the best motor response measured at any one limb. Many painful stimuli have been tried with nail bed pressure or sternal rub being two of the more frequently used.

It is important to note that someone who is dead is given a score of 3 on this scale. Some centers remove withdrawal to pain from the tabulation and therefore have the score out of 14 instead of 15. If using this modification it is important to let other clinicians know that you have done so.

Dr. Navraj Singh Heran

The Glasgow Coma scale is the foundation for how medical students, residents, practicing physicians, nurses, and even emergency health services communicate about a patient's neurologic status. It is simple, easy to memorize, simple to interpret, and readily documented and/or communicated.

As a practicing neurosurgeon, one of the major limitations of the scale is that it portrays only the best neurologic status of the patient. Therefore, a patient could be hemiplegic or paraplegic with no ability using the scale to communicate this information to those involved in caring for the patient. It is obvious, therefore, that in certain situations, particularly those of extra-axial hematomas, the system may not express the degree of potential danger the patient may be in.

For example, a patient who is opening eyes to speech, confused, and localizing on one side and flexor posturing on one side with a contralateral epidural hematoma, would score the same GCS numeric value as a patient with diffuse brain injury with the same neurologic findings but who is symmetrically localizing. Clearly, the first patient is in much more dire immediate situation yet the scale fails to demonstrate this. Therefore, in addition to the GCS score, I describe each side of the patient's motor assessment, therefore allowing subsequent or examiners comparing assessments to truly assess for changes.

On another note, I was not aware that some people exclude the withdrawal score. I do not quite understand why this is the case in these institutions as the difference between withdrawing and localizing may reflect only minimal discrepancies in sedation or degree of injury. It does appear to reflect the continuum among motor function within the scale although likely without the same degree of discrepancies as with the other motor scores.

Finally, the "ominpresent" rule of "GCS less than 8, intubate" is extremely simplistic and not applicable in various clinical scenarios. One such situation is a patient who sustains a craniocerebral injury that presents with a GCS less than 8 and who may have had an impact seizure. The majority of such patients will improve neurologically and therefore not require intubation and hence avoid the risks and resources associated with controlled airways and ventilation. In my opinion, the most important considerations in lower GCS score patients is the ABCs as based on vital sign monitoring, the direction the GCS score is trending, and the findings on cranial imaging.

High-Energy Ballistic and Avulsive Facial Injuries

What It Classifies

Soft tissue and bony injury to the face resulting from ballistic wounds (high energy) and the treatment of those injuries.

System

Etiology:

Gunshot (low and high velocity)

Rifle

Shotgun

Avulsive facial injuries

Regions of injury:

Lower midface and mandible

Infraorbital maxilla and occlusal areas

Orbit

Frontal bone and frontal sinus

The zones of tissue injury and tissue loss must be noted for each anatomic area. It is not necessary to define these injuries completely at the initial treatment, for a subsequent exploration confirms a high-energy injury by the pattern of evolving tissue necrosis.

Reference

Clark N, Birely B, Manson PN, et al. High-energy ballistic and avulsive facial injuries: classification, patterns, and an algorithm for primary reconstruction. *Plast Reconstr Surg.* 1996 (suppl 1);98(4):583–601.

Uses

Primary: Etiology, Description, Diagnosis, Treatment

Secondary: Research, Prognosis

Limited/none:

Comments

Dr. Paul Oxley

This classification is based on a 17-year review of fire arm and high-energy avulsive facial injuries (Fig 8–5). It is the first to include avulsive injuries as a ballistic or high-energy wound. High-energy avulsive wounds are described as those where the soft tissue has been extensively torn, crushed, and partially avulsed, rendering some areas ischemic. It is an anatomic and energy-based injury classification leading to an algorithm for the treatment of facial injury from the time of initial assessment to final reconstruction.

Four patterns for gunshot wounds and three for avulsive injuries were realized. Whereas gunshot wounds are best classified by the location of the exit wound, shotgun and avulsive facial wounds are classified according to the zone of soft-tissue and bone loss. Treatment, prognosis, and complications vary according to four patterns of gunshot wounds and four patterns of shotgun wounds.

The study showed that 76% of patients could be included in the above four patterns; therefore it has some limitations when describing the pattern of injury. It allows the surgeon to divide the areas

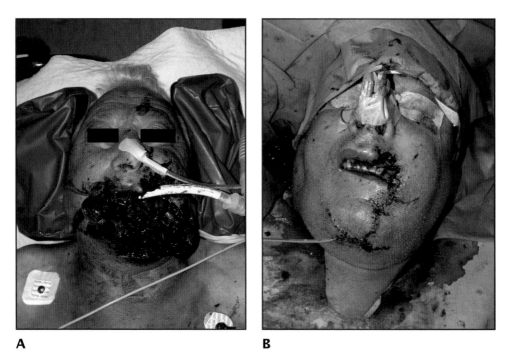

A   **B**

Fig 8–5. Facial gun shot wound with shot gun. **A.** Before and **B.** after debridement.

of the face and determine the injury and needs for each one. Prognosis is not specifically defined by level of energy, etiology, or anatomic location, but rather depends on a mixture of all three.

Dr. Oleh Antonyshyn

Massive compound injuries to the face causing both soft tissue and skeletal disruption are rare. Multiple disciplines are frequently involved in the care of these patients. The anatomic extent and degree of disruption may be difficult to determine

reliably following the first assessment, and multiple operative interventions are generally required. For all these reasons, high-energy ballistic and avulsive facial injuries have defied classification in the past.

This classification system is based on the experience gained in managing over 300 such injuries over a period of 15 years. The classification is based on both the etiology and the anatomic site of the injury. It is particularly useful in that it characterizes the degree of soft tissue and bony disruption and provides a guide to the reconstructive requirements.

Le Fort Classification

What It Classifies

Midface fractures.

System

I: Transverse maxillary fracture above alveolar process
II: Pyramidal fracture through maxilla, orbits, and frontonasal junction
III: Craniofacial disjunction

See Figure 8-6.

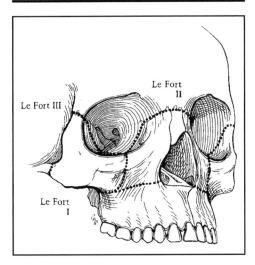

Fig 8–6. Le Fort fractures. Manson PN, Facial Fractures. In: Aston SJ, Beasley RW, Thorne CHM, eds, *Grabb and Smith's Plastic Surgery*, 5th ed. Philadelphia, Pa: Lippincott-Raven Publishers; 1997:383. Copyright 1997 by Lippincott, Williams & Wilkins. Reprinted with permission.

References

Le Fort R. Etude experimentale sur les fractures de la machorie superieure. *Rev Chir Paris.* 1901;208:479.

Manson PN. Facial fractures. In: Aston SJ, Beasley RW, Thorne CHM, eds. *Grabb and Smith's Plastic Surgery.* 5th ed. Philadelphia, Pa: Lippincott-Raven Publishers; 1997:383.

Uses

Primary: Description, Diagnosis

Secondary: Research, Treatment

Limited/none: Prognosis, Etiology

Comments

Dr. Paul Oxley

The origins of this classification system is one of the best stories in plastic surgery. Rene Le Fort conducted a series of experiments looking at the patterns of midfacial fractures, which are detailed in his 1901 paper. It is hard to imagine anyone getting ethical permission to redo these studies today. Each experiment consisted of a cadaver or cadaveric head being dropped, thrown, or hit with various objects, and the resulting fracture pattern analyzed. He determined three common patterns of midfacial fracture, and these are known eponymously as Le Fort I, II, or III.

Unfortunately, these fractures rarely happen in isolation or as pure injuries. The experiments were done with relatively low force, blunt trauma. Given the high-speed mechanisms seen today versus 100 years ago, it is uncommon to see the isolated injuires. A patient can have a Le Fort I on the right and a Le Fort II on the left, or a combined I and II on the same side. The term "hemi-Le Fort" is sometimes used to describe a one-sided injury. "High" and "low" are often used to modify Le Fort I designation with respect to its involvement of the piriform aperture. In addition, any other injuries, such as orbital floor blowout or alveolar fractures are described separately.

However, this classification system is widely used and understood, and best describes the midfacial fracture lines rather than the direction of fracture and bones involved. Treatment and prognosis depends on the severity of fractures and degree of asymmetry and displacement.

Dr. Oleh Antonyshyn

The Le Fort classification of midface fractures is based on an anatomic description of observed fracture patterns which occurred in cadaver experiments. These fracture patterns correspond to areas of relative weakness in the midfacial buttresses when direct frontal impact forces are applied.

This midfacial fracture classification is so widely accepted that anyone practicing facial reconstructive surgery must be familiar with it.

However, it is important to note the following: The classification is not comprehensive. Additional fracture patterns are frequently observed, particularly when applied forces are more localized, or when they are oriented in more vertically oriented directions. Therefore, a Le Fort classification of midfacial fractures should be supplemented with the following:

A classification of palatal fractures. Palatal fractures were described and classified by Hendrickson M, Clarke M, and Manson PN et al in *Plastic and Reconstructive Surgery,* 1998;101(2):319 to 332. They are classified as:

  i. anterior and posterolateral alveolar
 ii. sagittal
iii. parasagittal
 iv. para-alveolar
  v. complex
 vi. transverse

It is also extremely important to note that although Le Fort I, II, and III patterns are consistently observed in midfacial fractures, they are not generally seen in isolation. This is particularly true in high-velocity massive impact injuries. Under these circumstances, it is much more common to see fracture lines at multiple levels corresponding to Le Fort I, II, and III patterns. For example, a patient might present with a right Le Fort III, II, I, and a left Le Fort I fracture.

Mandible Fractures

What It Classifies

Stability of mandible fractures based on location and the direction of muscle pull.

System

Favorable:

Nondisplaced by muscle pull

Stable fractures

Most ramus fractures

Angle fractures extending superiorly to inferiorly as it extends anteriorly

Unfavorable:

Horizontally unfavorable

Angle fractures extending posteriorly and downward

Due to muscles of mastication

Vertically unfavorable

Symphyseal

Parasymphyseal

Due to action of suprahyoid muscles

Laterally unfavorable

High condylar fractures

Medially displaced due to lateral pterygoid muscle

See Figure 8-7.

References

Clark N. Mandibular fractures. In: Georgiade GS, Riefkohl R, Levin LS, eds. *Georgiade Plastic, Maxillofacial and Reconstructive Surgery.* Baltimore, Md: Williams and Wilkins; 1997:377-405.

Stacey DH, Doyle JF, Mount DL, Snyder MC, Gutowski KA. Management of mandible fractures. *Plast Reconstr Surg.* 2006; 117(3):48e-60e.

Uses

Primary: Description

Secondary: Treatment, Prognosis, Research, Diagosis

Limited/none: Etiology

Comments

Dr. Paul Oxley

Fractures of the mandible can be classified in many different ways:

Open or closed

Simple, comminuted or greenstick

Location on the mandible

Unilateral or bilateral

Stable or unstable

Location next to teeth

Size of remaining mandible in the edentulous mandible

This system denotes a fracture as either inherently stable or unstable, and from this determination, management is easily extrapolated. Although stable fractures can theoretically be left alone or managed with a minor operation, unstable

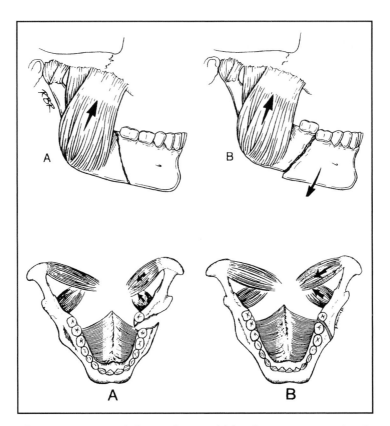

Fig 8–7. Favorability of Mandible fractures. **A** (*top*): Unfavorable angle-body fracture. **B** (*top*): favorable fracture. **A** (*bottom*): unfavorable angle, and **B** (*bottom*): favorable fracture location. Clark N. Mandibular fractures. In: Georgiade GS, Riefkohl R, Levin LS, eds. *Georgiade Plastic, Maxillofacial and Reconstructive Surgery.* Baltimore, Md: Williams and Wilkins; 1997:377–405. Copyright 1997 by Lippincott, Williams & Wilkins. Reprinted with permission.

fractures always require operative intervention to obtain a satisfactory result. There are many different methods used to repair a fracture and maintain normal occlusion.

Dr. Robyn Watts

Several muscles act on the mandible. As a result of these differing forces, frac-ture segments are commonly displaced depending on the location and orientation of the fracture. There are two main groups of muscles that act on the mandible including the muscles of mastication and the suprahyoid muscles. The muscles of mastication include the masseter, temporalis, and the medial and lateral pterygoid muscles. The suprahyoid muscles include the digastric, stylohyoid, mylohyoid, and geniohyoid muscles. The muscles of mastication tend to pull posterior segments superiorly whereas the suprahyoid muscles tend to pull the anterior segments inferiorly. The lateral pterygoids tend to pull the condylar head medially.

Fractures of the mandible have been classified in many ways such as by anatomic location, whether or not they are displaced, comminuted, open or closed, stable or unstable. The above classification attempts to classify fractures based on both anatomic locations and the direction of muscle pull resulting in either a favorable or unfavorable fracture. The advantage of this classification is that it not only describes the location of the fracture but also its inherent stability and whether or not surgical management is likely required. It does not, however, give any information as to how each different fracture should be managed. In addition, this classification does not delineate open versus closed fractures nor simple versus comminuted fractures which is important information when deciding on management. It is a useful descriptive classification, however, like most, it has its limitations.

Dr. Kevin L. Bush

This classification of mandible fractures is based on the stability of mandible fractures as determined by the angle of the fracture and the associated pull of the muscles of mastication. It is an older classification which was of good use during the time when rigid fixation was not available or the risks of rigid fixation were significant.

Application of this classification of mandible fractures would indeed influence clinical decisions applied to the treatment of mandible fractures. However, I feel it is no longer of real significance in today's clinical use simply because the widespread use of open reduction internal fixation of many mandible fractures makes the diagnosis of a favorable versus unfavorable fracture based on the location of fracture pattern and muscle pull less relevant.

An anatomic classification is much more useful in terms of describing the mandible fracture and directing communication between physicians. The anatomic classification also directs the physician to a number of choices available for specific fractures regardless of whether the fracture is favorable or unfavorable.

Nasal Deviation

What It Classifies

Anatomic patterns producing nasal deviation.

System

  I. Caudal septal deviation
    a. Straight septal tilt
    b. Concave deformity
    c. S-shaped deformity
  II. Concave dorsal deformity
    a. C-shaped dorsal deformity
    b. Reverse C-shaped dorsal deformity
  III. Concave/convex dorsal deformity
    (S-shaped)

Reference

Rohrich RJ, Gunter JP, Deuber MA, Adams WP Jr. The deviated nose: optimizing results using a simplified classification and algorithmic approach. *Plast Reconstr Surg.* 2002;110(6):1509–1523.

Uses

Primary: Description, Diagnosis, Treatment

Secondary: Research, Treatment

Limited/none: Etiology, Prognosis

Comments

Dr. Paul Oxley

In rhinoplasty the surgeon must define the parts of the nasal appearance that are of concern to the patient and whether or not these can be predictably corrected. As each nose is different and each individual has different ideas as to what is an aesthetically pleasing nose, this is an important factor in performing a successful rhinoplasty and having a satisfied patient. Nasal deviation can combine both a functional (airway) and aesthetic problem.

Rohrich and colleagues present an approach to the deviated nose using preoperative planning and intraoperative techniques. The key points of this anatomic scheme are the maintenance of dorsal aesthetic lines and a patent airway via an open and systematic approach. These techniques are well described in the original paper.

The authors divide nasal deviation into three main groups, focusing on the anatomy of the nasal dorsum and caudal septum. Deviation of the septum may or may not effect the outer appearance of the nose, but will have an effect on the passage of air. The most common deformity is type Ia. Concavity of the dorsum is the most common external cause of the deviated nose.

This classification is very useful for identifying and planning surgical correction of nasal deviation. It is easy to apply, and though it does not grade each specific deformity, it provides corrective techniques regardless of severity. It is important to remember that each nose is individual and end results will vary by the starting position. The system is also useful in research as it clearly describes a problem and is easily reproduced.

Dr. Oleh Antonyshyn

Classification systems are particularly useful when they serve to guide decision-making during the evaluation or treatment of a clinical problem. The classification of nasal deviation proposed by Rohrich, Gunter, et al, accomplishes this very effectively. The surgeon must assess the degree of caudalseptal deviation and dorsal septal deviation separately. The specific techniques that are effective in reconstructing caudal and dorsal septal deviations, respectively, are then described.

The classification is perhaps overly detailed in describing the direction of deviation. Whether the septum is deviated with a concavity to the left or to the right is irrelevant to the final treatment. Simi-larly, whether the deviation is C-shaped or S-shaped simply describes the direction of deflection and does not affect decisions regarding treatment.

I would suggest that nasal deviations could be more simply classified according to the treatment algorithm proposed by the authors in this very same article. Specifically, a nasal deviation can be classified as:

1. Caudalseptal deviation
   a. Straight septal tilt
   b. Curved deformity
2. Dorsal septal deviation.

Nasal Fractures

What It Classifies

Patterns of fracture of the nose.

AKA

Stranc and Robertson Nasal Fracture Classification

System

Plane 1: Disruption of the cartilage, nasal bones unaffected.

Plane 2: Disruption of the bony septum and nasal bones.

Plane 3: Extension beyond nasal skeleton to piriform aperture and orbital rim.

See Figure 8–8.

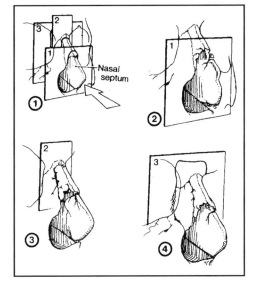

Fig 8–8. Nasal fractures. Manson PN. The management of midfacial and frontal bone fractures. In: Georgiade GS, Riefkohl R, Levin LS, eds. *Georgiade Plastic, Maxillofacial and Reconstructive Surgery.* Baltimore, Md: Williams and Wilkins; 1997:356. Copyright 1997 by Lippincott, Williams & Wilkins. Reprinted with permission.

References

Manson PN. The management of midfacial and frontal bone fractures. In: Georgiade GS, Riefkohl R, Levin LS, eds. *Georgiade Plastic, Maxillofacial and Reconstructive Surgery.* Baltimore, Md: Williams and Wilkins; 1997:356

Stranc MF, Robertson GA. A classification of injuries of the nasal skeleton. *Ann Plast Surg.* 1978;2:468.

Uses

Primary: Diagnosis, Description, Treatment

Secondary: Research

Limited/none: Etiology, Prognosis

Comments

Dr. Paul Oxley

Most nasal fractures can be described as pushed to one side (deviated), pushed posteriorly, a combination of the two, or undisplaced. As most nasal fractures are described by these anatomic terms, the above system is not widely used.

This system does include the extent of injury beyond the simple anatomic distortion. By so doing, it is much more useful in research, looking at different causes and treatments of nasal fractures. However, it does not directly describe the severity or direction of the fracture, which can strongly influence treatment options and prognosis.

Dr. Nick Carr

In reviewing this classification, the treatment and implications of the fracture should be included. In plane 1 it may be difficult to correct primarily and may require secondary septorhinoplasty. In plane 2 it is important to attempt accurate primary reduction whereas in plane 3, CT evaluation is important and the fracture may require open reduction and fixation.

In all, this is not a terribly useful classification in that the majority of nasal fractures can be treated without consideration of this, that is, to reduce primarily based on clinical appearance. Secondary septorhinoplasty is then considered if necessary

Naso-orbito-ethmoidal Complex Fractures

What It Classifies

Fractures of the naso-orbito-ethmoidal (NOE) region.

System

I: Complete or incomplete fracture, single fragment.
    IA: Incomplete fracture, single fragment
    IB: Complete fracture, single fragment
    IC: Complete fracture, bilateral monobloc
II: Comminuted fractures external to the canthal insertion
III: Comminuted fractures extending within the canthal insertion

See Figure 8–9.

Reference

Grant MP, Iliff NT, Manson PN. Naso-orbito-ethmoidal complex injuries. In: Evans GRD, ed. *Operative Plastic Surgery.* New York, NY: McGraw-Hill;2000:575.

Uses

Primary: Description, Diagnosis, Treatment

Secondary: Prognosis, Research

Limited/none: Etiology

Comments

Dr. Paul Oxley

This classification is designed to help direct treatment and surgical approach based on fracture pattern. The basis of the system is the fracture pattern, the position of the central medial canthal bearing bone fragment, the presence of fractures at its distal articulations, and the presence of internal fractures, especially at the insertion point of the canthal ligaments. The classification addresses only fractures of the NOE, and does not include those associated with other facial fractures.

Basically, treatment is determined by the position and integrity of the canthal insertion and the ability to reduce and stabilize the bony injury.

This system is easy to use and leaves little open to subjective interpretation. Specific treatment does depend on clinical experience as well as the presence of other injuries. Prognosis depends as much on time to treatment, experience of the surgeon, and other related injuries as it does to specific NOE fracture pattern.

Dr. Oleh Antonyshyn

This classification of naso-orbitoethmoidal fractures was first described by Marke-witz, Manson and Sergeant, et al in 1991 (*Plastic and Reconstructive Surgery.* 1991;87(5):843–853).

This classification system is one of the best examples of a classification system that can be simple and yet readily applicable in virtually all clinical situations. This classification system is the most basic and fundamental guide to identifying, diagnosing and treating naso-orbitoethmoidal injuries.

The classification system is based on the degree of disruption of the "central" fragment: that is, the segment of the

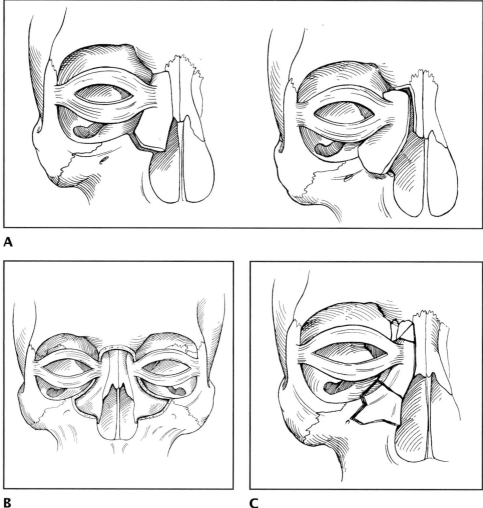

Fig 8–9. NOE Fractures: **A.** Type I fractures. (*Left*), incomplete type 1A "green-stick" fracture. In this fracture, there is no displacement superiorly at internal angular process of frontal bone; however, there is fracture with displacement at inferior orbital rim and pyriform aperture. (*Right*), complete type 1B fracture. Complete fractures have inferior displacement at internal angular process of frontal bone and inferiorly at inferior orbital rim and piriform aperature. Fracture requires operative treatment at three locations. In incomplete fracture, displacement may be corrected by approaches to only inferior fractures. **B.** Type IC, Monoblock NOE fracture (complete bilateral monoblock). Fracture results in one-piece bilateral fracture that isolates single bony fragment containing insertions of both medial canthi. As bone continuity is retained across midline, telecanthus is not possible. **C.** Type II complete fracture. Type II fractures may be either unilateral or bilateral; unilateral fracture is shown. Note that fracture is comminuted external to insertion of medial canthal tendon. Proper identification and management of "central fragment" during dissection and fixation are critical aspects of facture treatment. *continues*

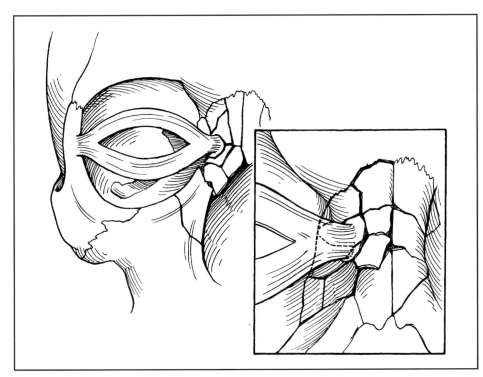

D

Fig 8–9. *continued* **D.** Type III fracture. Type III fracture is defined as complete fracture with comminution of central fragment or tendon avulsion. In these situations, transnasal reduction of canthal realignment is necessary in addition to reduction of bony frontal process of maxilla. Grant MP, Iliff NT, Manson PN. Naso-orbito-ethmoidal complex injuries. In: *Operative Plastic Surgery*, Evans GRD, ed. New York, NY: McGraw-Hill;2000,:575. Copyright 2000 by The McGraw-Hill Companies. Reprinted with permission.

medial orbital rim which contains the insertion of the medial canthal tendon. Clinically, use of this classification system necessitates a very thorough clinical and radiologic assessment which identifies the following:

1. a fracture circumscribing the "*central*" fragment
2. the presence or absence of displacement of this "*central*" fragment
3. the degree of disruption, that is, the degree of comminution and/or

bone loss in the surrounding bone of the frontal process of the maxilla, the nasal process of the frontal bone, nose, and medial orbital wall.

Once a patient's fracture pattern is identified and characterized according to this classification, the approach to surgical reconstruction, in terms of the type of exposure needed, the fixation requirements and the possible need for bone grafting, is greatly simplified.

Palatal Fractures

What It Classifies

Fractures of the palate with modifiers for soft tissue lacerations.

AKA

Hendrickson System

System

Type I: Alveolar—Anterior and/or posterolateral

Type II: Sagittal—Along midpalatal suture from piriform aperture

Type III: Parasagittal—Along the thinner bone lateral to the vomerine attachment extending from between the cuspid teeth, piriform aperture, and may track along the midline or extend laterally toward the tuberosity

Type IV: Para-alveolar—Medial to the maxillary alveolus

Type V: Complex—dividing the palate obliquely and transversely, or comminuting the palate and alveolus

Type VI: Transverse—divides the palate and maxilla in a coronal plane

Modify for laceration:

A: None

B: Simple

C: Complex

Reference

Hendrickson M, Clark N, Manson PN, et al. Palatal fractures: classification, patterns, and treatment with rigid internal fixation. *Plast Reconstr Surg.* 1998;101(2):319-332.

Uses

Primary: Description, Diagnosis, Treatment

Secondary: Research

Limited/none: Prognosis, Etiology

Comments

Dr. Rizwan Mian and Dr. Paul Oxley

Palatal fractures can be very difficult to correct. Obtaining normal occlusion is paramount in treating these injuries. They are present in roughly 8% of Le Fort fractures, or can be an isolated fracture in the absence of other Le Fort pattern injuries. It is crucial to understand the scope of the injury prior to treatment.

In addition to developing the above classification, this study also showed that rigid internal fixation of these fractures reduces the time spent in intermaxillary fixation (IMF). The classification was created using CT images of fractures.

It is a very simple classification and clearly describes the clinical problem. By correlating the fracture pattern to treatment in the original article, it makes this a very useful classification for any surgeon dealing with these injuries. It facilitates treatment decisions and would help plan studies.

Nevertheless, this classification is often not used on a regular basis in the clinical setting and is not particularly useful to the average clinician.

Treatment of Palatal Fractures

What It Classifies

Palatal fractures based on surgical treatment.

System

1. Closed reduction type
   - Undisplaced alveolar fracture
   - Includes many Hendrickson type I
2. Anterior type
   - Only anterior surface of maxilla exposed
   - Rigid fixation on maxillary buttress, alveolar ridge, ± piriform rim
   - Includes some Hendrickson type I, IV, and VI
3. Anterior and palatal type
   - Sagittally split palate large enough to plate
   - Differs from #2 above by presence of large palatal fracture fragments
   - Usually includes Hendrickson's type II and III
4. Combined type
   - Severe comminution or missing bone.
   - Requires ORIF and IMF
   - Includes some Hendrickson type IV, V, and VI

Reference

Park S, Ock JJ. A new classification of palatal fracture and an algorithm to establish a treatment plan. *Plast Reconstr Surg.* 2001; 107(7):1669-1676.

Uses

Primary: Treatment

Secondary: Description, Diagnosis

Limited/none: Etiology, Prognosis, Research

Comments

Dr. Paul Oxley

Like most injuries, there are many ways of classifying palatal fractures. They can be looked at from the point of view of Description, Diagnosis, Etiology, or Treatment. The primary classification system for fractured palates (Hendrickson) describes the fracture line and fragment positions. The authors have attempted to take the classification one step further by looking at how fractures should be managed.

It takes a basic understanding of fracture patterns and treatment options to understand this classification. The system is designed to help identify the correct treatment for any given fracture. However, although it may simplify the surgical options for these fractures, most occur in association with other significant facial fractures. Therefore, other options for any given fracture may need to be considered. For example, in the presence of a mandibular fracture, IMF may be required even though this classification only calls for ORIF.

Dr. Robyn Watts

Like many fractures, there are many ways to describe palatal fractures. Hendrickson et al attempted to do so by describing the anatomic location of the fracture line and fragment position in types I to VI. In the above classification, Park et al have taken this one step further by establishing a treatment algorithm for each of their subclassifications. They have at-tempted to describe a treatment plan and surgical approach based on each subtype which is useful in so far as deciding on a course of action and in learning the treatment principles of these challenging and rare facial fractures. Unfortunately, this classification is less descriptive and makes it more difficult to both remember and interpret especially when it comes to teaching young surgeons.

I think that this classification would be most useful when combined with Hendrickson's classification in that it both describes the anatomic location and fracture pattern, along the appropriate treatment plan. This undoubtedly makes the classification more complicated, however, more complete.

Zygoma Fractures

What It Classifies

Zygoma fracture patterns.

AKA

Knight and North Classification of Zygoma Fractures

System

   I: Undisplaced fractures (6%)
  II: Displaced arch fracture (10%)
 III: Displaced body fracture with no rotation (33%)

 IV: Displaced body fracture with medial rotation (11%)
  V: Displaced body fracture with lateral rotation (22%)
 VI: Complex fracture (18%)

See Figure 8–10.

References

Knight JS, North JF. The classification of malar fractures: an analysis of displacement as a guide to treatment. *Br J Plast Surg.* 1961; 13:325–339.

Manson PN. Facial fractures. In: Aston SJ, Beasley RW, Thorne CHM, eds. *Grabb and Smith's Plastic Surgery.* 5th ed. Philadelphia, Pa: Lippincott-Raven Publishers; 1997:391.

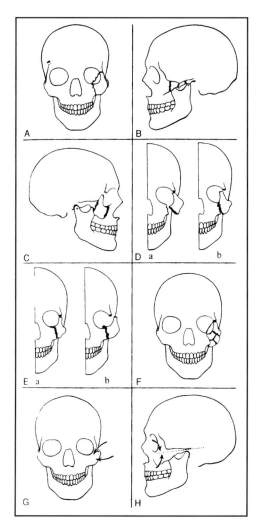

Fig 8–10. Zygoma fractures. Manson PN, Facial Fractures. In: Aston SJ, Beasley RW, Thorne CHM, eds, *Grabb and Smith's Plastic Surgery*, 5th ed. Philadelphia, Pa: Lippincott-Raven Publishers; 1997:391. Copyright 1997 by Lippincott, Williams & Wilkins. Reprinted with permission.

Uses

Primary: Description, Diagnosis, Research

Secondary: Treatment

Limited/none: Etiology, Prognosis

Comments

Dr. Paul Oxley

This is a very comprehensive classification and yet it is not widely used. It is slightly outdated in that the distribution of fractures described in the study will have changed due to the changing sources of facial fractures in society. The percentages will vary depending on mechanism. The classification does not take into account other fractures and therefore has little predictive ability with respect to prognosis. Similarly, treatment options are more related to degree of displacement and the presence of other injuries. There is no place in this classification for describing a concomitant orbital floor fracture, as it is generally believed that all zygoma fractures will have some component of orbital floor involvement.

Dr. Robyn Watts

Zygomatic fractures, albeit one of the most common traumatic facial injuries seen by plastic surgeons, remain a difficult problem for students to conceptualize. It is important to first understand the complex three-dimensional structure of the zygomatic bone and its interfaces prior to conceptualizing the outcomes of trauma such as fracture pattern and possible orientation of the displaced bone.

The classification by Knight and North is widely used to describe zygomatic fractures by taking into account fracture location in addition to displacement and orientation of the bony fragment. It is an easy classification to interpret and simple enough to remember. It is useful in that it takes into account the location of the fracture such as arch versus body fractures and includes a subclassification for complex or comminuted fractures. It is also helpful in surgical planning as it delineates between those fractures that can be treated conservatively (undisplaced) versus those requiring surgical intervention (displaced). By further dividing displaced fractures into arch and body fractures with no rotation, medial rotation, and lateral rotation, this system helps the surgeon decide on an approach to surgery. The isolated medially displaced arch fracture is generally reduced with an elevator passed through a temporal approach, whereas the laterally displaced arch may require a coronal incision and arch reduction.

Unfortunately, this classification does not take into account the integrity of the orbital floor nor does it describe inward versus outward displacement of the components of the bony orbit which may affect the urgency to surgically treat a specific injury.

Chapter 9

VASCULAR MALFORMATIONS AND HEMANGIOMAS

Schobinger Classification

What It Classifies

Arteriovenous malformations.

AKA

Schobinger Staging System

System

Stage I: Blue skin blush/stain, warmth and AV shunting by continuous Doppler or 20-MHz color Doppler

Stage II: Same as Stage I, plus enlargement, tortuous tense veins, pulsations, bruit, and/or thrill

Stage III: Same as above, plus either dystrophic changes,

ulceration, bleeding, persistent pain, or destruction

Stage IV: Same as Stage II plus cardiac failure

Reference

Mulliken JB. Vascular anomalies. In: Aston SJ, Beasley RW, Thorne CHM, eds. *Grabb and Smith's Plastic Surgery*. 5th ed. Philadelphia, Pa; Lippincott-Raven Publishers; 1997:191.

Uses

Primary: Diagnosis, Research

Secondary: Prognosis, Description, Treatment

Limited/none: Etiology

Comments

Dr. Paul Oxley

This classification documents the evaluation of arteriovenous malformations from a primarily clinical point of view, taking into account ultrasonographic or Doppler findings. Each progressive level indicates an increased degree of severity, and a worsening prognosis. As it does not indicate the size or possible mass effect of the lesion it is not a clear or precise descriptive tool. Specific treatment is not implied for each level. The location and size of the arteriovenous malformation have a significant impact on the treatment choices.

Dr. Doug Courtemanche

This classification was derived and accepted at an early meeting of the International Society for Study of Vascular Anomalies (ISSVA). It is probably first referenced by Enjolras. It has never been published as a stand-alone paper with the reasons for the definitions of the various stages of degeneration in AVMs.

It is of historic interest and represents a step in the understanding of the evolution of pathologic changes in AVMs. There are few papers that use this classification to document patients with AVMs and relate the classification scheme to treatment decisions and outcomes. There is little information as to the timecourse of the progression of AVMs through the various stages and it is not clear that they all do. Most modern Vascular Anomalies Clinics would favor early intervention for AVMs due to the risk of progression and the increasing difficulty in treating lesions at a higher stage.

Vascular Anomalies of Infancy and Childhood

What It Classifies

All vascular lesions including tumours and malformations.

System

See Table 9–1.

Table 9–1. Vascular Anomalies

Tumors
Common
Infantile hemangiomas
Uncommon
Kaposiform hemangioendothelioma
Tufted angioma
Congenital hemangiopericytoma
Epithelioid hemangioma/ hemangioendothelioma
Angiosarcoma
Malformations
Slow-Flow
Capillary (CM): telangectasias
Lymphatic (LM)
Venous (VM)
Fast-Flow
Arterial (AM): aneurysm, coarctaton, ectasia, stenosis
Arteriovenous fistula (AVF)
Arteriovenous malformation (AVM)
Combined Malformations
Klippel-Trenaunay Syndrome (CLVM)
Parkes-Weber Syndrome (CLAVM, CLAVF)

References

Mulliken JB. Vascular anomalies. In: Aston SJ, Beasley RW, Thorne CHM, eds. *Grabb and Smith's Plastic Surgery.* 5th ed. Philadelphia, Pa: Lippincott-Raven Publishers; 1997:191.

Marler JJ, Mulliken JB. Current management of hemangiomas and vascular malformations, *Clin Plast Surg.* 2005;32(1):99–116.

Uses

Primary: Research, Description, Diagnosis, Etiology

Secondary: Treatment, Prognosis

Limited/none:

Comments

Dr. Paul Oxley

Originally presented in 1982 by Mulliken and Glowacki, this binary system of classifying vascular anomalies as tumors or malformations has greatly simplified our understanding of these lesions. It is the official classification of the International Society for the Study of Vascular Anomalies. It is very comprehensive, allowing for easy use in research, description, and diagnosis. Any student trying to understand vascular tumours and malformations should study from this table and try to avoid outdated terms for different lesions. Unfortunately, terms like "port-wine stain" and "cavernous hemangioma" are still used (Fig 9–1).

Some still lump all these together under the term "hemangioma," which is histologically incorrect and confuses

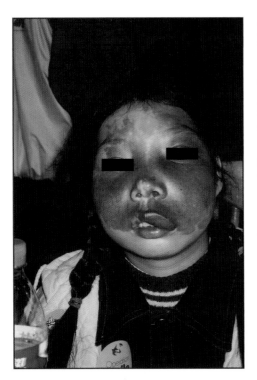

Fig 9–1. Large slow-flow capillary malformation.

students. This classification directs therapy and predicts prognosis. For example, macrocystic lymphatic malformations are often treated with sclerotherapy, whereas microcystic lesions require surgical resection. However, treatment and prognosis of any given lesion will also depend on location, size, and concomitant illness.

Dr. Luis Vasconez

Lumping together tumors as well as vascular malformations in the category of "Hemangiomas" has no prognostic value and does not help us in the treatment of these lesions.

Mulliken's attempt to categorize and classify these lesions is most worthwhile. Although it is clear that capillary, venous, and lymphatic malformations are indicative of the predominance of each particular vascular tissue, there are combined lesions such as lymphatic venous and particularly the most troublesome arteriovenous malformations (Fig 9–2).

The classification implies, but falls short on indicating prognosis. For example, most infantile hemangiomas will involute prior to puberty. Venous malformations are amenable to sclerosing agents and/or excision if they are relatively well circumscribed. It is less clear whether lymphatic malformations involute at least partially, and usually require surgical resection. Finally, arteriovenous malformations are presently ameliorated by super selective embolization or sclerotherapy; sometimes they can be resected.

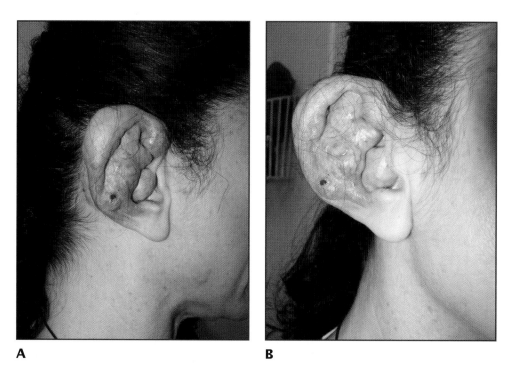

A

B

Fig 9–2. Arteriovenous malformation of the ear. **A.** Lateral view **B.** Anterior oblique view.

TERMS

Acrocephaly: Bilateral coronal suture synostoses. High skull.

Acrofacial Dydostosis: Aka Nager Syndrome.

Albinism: Hypopigmentation of skin, eyes, hair with high rate of SCC and BCC.

Albright disease: Polyostotic fibrous dysplasia, precocious puberty, café-au-lait lesions, and tumors of the pituitary gland.

Angel kiss: Aka Salmon patch, Stork bite. Macular patch on the posterior neck seen inover 50% of newborns. Flat, pale pink to brown, fade slowly.

Anotia: Complete failure of development of the auricular helix through a lack of mesenchymal proliferation

Apert syndrome: (Previously known as Acrocephalosyndactyly type I). Coronal and sphenoparietal squamosal synostoses. Mental retardation common. Turribrachycephaly, high steep and flat occiput and forehead with transverse forehead groove, midface hypoplasia with class III malocclusion, orbital hypertelorism with exorbitism, acne vulgaris, occasional cleft palate (30%), synbrachydactyly. Autosomal dominant.

Auriculotemporal nerve syndrome: Aka Frey syndrome. Gustatory sweating following facelift.

Bands of Buengner: Bands formed by collapsed columns of nerve cells on electron microscopy after nerve injury.

Basal cell nevus syndrome: Aka Gorlin syndrome. Three key findings: Multiple BCC's, jaw cysts (odontogenic keratocysts), pitting of palms and soles. Other findings: pseudohypertelorism, frontal bossing, syndactyly, spina bifida.

Baze-Dupre-Christol syndrome: X-linked with follicular atrophoderma, congenital hypotrichosis, basal cell nevi and BCC.

Bazek syndrome: Multiple BCCs with follicular atrophoderma.

Bean syndrome: Aka Blue rubber bleb syndrome.

Becker nevus: Dark patch on the shoulder, appears during adolescence, may become hairy.

Beckwith-Weidemann syndrome: Unknown etiology. Gaping mouth, macroglossia, and prognathism. Large body size, umbilical hernia or omphalocele, neonatal hypoglycemia, metopic synostoses. May be associated with Wilm's tumor (kidney), seizure disorders, and high aspiration risk.

Bell's palsy: Idiopathic facial nerve paralysis.

Bell's phenomenon: Protective upward movement of the globe on closure of the eyelids.

Binder syndrome: Aka maxillonasal dysplasia. Mid facial hypoplasia with decreased vertical height of maxilla, short and flat nose, short or absent columella, absent anterior nasal spine, normal intelligence, 50% vertebral anomalies. Fossa prenasalis present.

Blue rubber bleb syndrome: Aka Bean syndrome. Multiple venous malformations of hands, feet, and GI tract.

Blue spot: Dermal melanocytosis causing blue-gray discolouration over the sacrum.

Bowen disease: Intraepithelial SCC (SCC in situ).

Boxy nasal tip: Broad, rectangular appearance of the tip lobule on basal view.

Brachycephaly: Bilateral coronal synostoses (also causes turricephaly and acrocephaly) or bilateral lambdoid suture synostoses. Short skull anteroposteriorly. Commonly seen in Apert's and Crouzon's syndromes.

Café-au-lait patch: Light brown epidermal melanocytic patch.

Calcifying epithelioma of Malherbe: Aka pilomatrixoma. Hard subcutaneous nodule arising from hair follicles.

Campbell de Morgan spots: AV fistula at the dermal capillary level seen in sun-exposed areas and with aging.

Carpenter syndrome: Aka Acrocephalopolysyndactyly. Variable synostoses. Tower skull, down thrust eyes, orbital hypertelorism with exorbitism, low-set ears, high and narrow arched palate. Also obesity, hypogonadism, D3, 4 syndactyly, preaxial polydactyly, ventricular septal defect (VSD), atrial septal defect (ASD), and mental retardation. Autosomal recessive.

Cherubism: Familial fibrous dysplasia, polysostotic of mandible and maxilla, self-limiting.

Cloverleaf skull deformity: Aka Kleeblattschadel.

Cobb syndrome: Truncal capillary malformation with underlying spinal AVM.

Coloboma: Missing segment of an eyelid causing a gap.

Cowden syndrome: Multiple facial tricholemmomas, keratoses on the palms and soles, oral polyps. 50% of patients will develop breast cancer. Alleleic with Bannazin-Riley-Ruvalcaba syndrome (PTEN mutation).

Craniofacial microsomia: Aka hemifacial microsomia or 1st and 2nd "branchial" arch syndrome.

Crouzon syndrome: Aka Craniofacial dysostosis. Coronal and sometimes saggital suture synostoses. Autosomal dominant, sporadic. Occasional minor mental deficiency. Tower skull, orbital hypertelorism with exorbitism, midfacial hypoplasia with class III malocclusion, beaked nose, and high, arched palate.

Crumpled ear: Folded-over appearance. Ridging is present along the helical rim, the scapha, and the antihelix. The skin is also involved in the crumpled appearance. Often associated with Beal syndrome.

Cryptotia: Abnormal adherence of the ear to the temporal skin associated with cartilage malformation in the scapha-antihelix complex.

Cup ear: Malformed, protruding ear combining characteristics of both a lop ear and a prominent ear. Typically this includes an overdeveloped, deep, cup-shaped concha, a deficient superior part of the helical margin and crura, and small vertical height. The body of the antihelix is often wider than normal, exaggerating the defect.

Cutis aplasia: Absence of all layers of scalp with skull and dura involved in severe case.

Cutis laxa: Textured, drooping skin from neonatal period. Lack elastase inhibitor. Also have aneurysms, pneumothroaces, emphysema, hernias, and congenital heart disease. Normal wound healing.

Darwin tubercle: Tuberculum auriculae (ear).

DiGeorge association: Aka Velocardiofacial syndrome. Abnormalities of the immune system and calcium levels seen in 10% of patients with Shprintzen syndrome.

Down syndrome: Birth defects due to triple chromosome 21. Mental retardation of varying severity, low-set ears, epicanthic folds.

Ehlers-Danlos syndrome: Heterogeneous collection of connective tissue disorders due to defects in the synthesis, structure, or cross-linking of collagen. Mostly autosomal dominant except type II which is X-linked. Avoid surgery where possible. Hypermobile joints, distensible skin, easily bruised, fragile connective tissue, aortic aneurysms.

Epidermodysplasia verruciformis: Autosomal recessive, cell-mediated immunity disorder of several HPV subtypes that induce numerous polymorphic verrucous lesions with a high transformation rate to SCC.

Epidermolysis bullosa: Unusual susceptibility to mechanical stress on skin. Nikowsky sign. Dermatolytic bullous dermatosis leading to hand contractures.

Erythroplasia of Queyrat: Intraepithelial SCC (in situ SCC) affecting the mucous membranes, often affecting the glans penis and higher rates seen in the 5th and 6th decades. Also known as Bowen disease of the mucous membranes.

FAMM Flap: Facial artery musculomucosal flap.

Ferguson disease: Aka Ferguson-Smith syndrome. Multiple self-healing keratoacanthomas. Autosomal dominant.

Fibrous Dysplasia: Abnormal proliferation of bone forming mesenchyme. Occurs in membranous bones of children. Lesions usually osseus not fibrous, monostotic more common than polyostotic.

Forme Fruste: General term often applied to microform cleft lips. A very minor form of incomplete cleft lip. May present as a minor depression in the alar cartilage, or a notch or depression along the philtral ridge.

Fossa prenasalis: Pit at inferior margin of piriform aperture. Seen in Binder association.

Franschetti syndrome: Aka Treacher Collins syndrome.

Frey syndrome: Aka auriculotemporal nerve syndrome. Gustatory sweating following facelift.

Gardener syndrome: Multiple epidermoid cysts associated with osteomas of the jaw and polyposis coli.

Geurin fracture: Aka Le Fort I fracture.

Giant congenital nevus: Congenital nevus encompassing 1% or more of total body surface area of the head or neck, or 2% or more of anywhere else on the body.

Glossoptosis: Large protruding tongue seen typically in Robin sequence.

Goldenhar syndrome: Alternate name for presentation of hemifacial microsomia with a classic triad of findings: Hemifacial Microsomia, epibulbar dermoids, vertebral abnormalities.

Gorham Stout disease: Aka missing bone disease. Lymphatic malformations with multiple areas of bone degeneration.

Gorlin syndrome: Aka Basal Cell Nevus syndrome. Three key findings: Multiple BCC's, jaw cysts (odontogenic keratocysts), pitting of palms and soles. Other findings: pseudohypertelorism, frontal bossing, syndactyly, spina bifida.

Harlequin deformity: Characteristic radiologic finding of patients with synostotic frontal plagiocephaly (unilateral coronal synostoses). It is an abnormal shape of the orbit due to ipsilateral superior displacement of the lesser wing of the sphenoid.

Hemifacial atrophy: Aka Romberg disease.

Hemifacial microsomia: Aka 1st and 2nd branchial arch syndrome. Congenital underdevelopment of one side of the face. OMENS (Orbit, Mandible, Ear, Nerve [CN VII] and Soft tissue) are all underdeveloped.

Holoprosencephalic disorders: A midline facial anomaly caused by either soft tissue volume deficiency or excess.

Horner syndrome: Ptosis, myosis, anhydrosis, ± enophthalmos due to loss of sympathetic tone.

Hutchinson freckle: Lentigo maligna melanoma. Invasive counterpart of lentigo maligna. May be very slow onset from time of development of lentigo maligna.

Hypertelorism: Excess distance between the orbits.

Jadassohn sebaceous nevus: *See* Nevus sebaceous of Jadassohn.

Juvenile melanoma: *See* Spitz nevus.

Kasabach-Merritt syndrome: DIC, thrombocytopenia, microangiopathic hemolytic anemia. Raised INR, PTT, and FDP. Low fibrinogen. Associated with Kaposiform hemangioendothelioma and tufted angioma.

Kleeblattschadel: Multiple or pansutural synostoses. Clover-leaf shaped skull.

Klippel-Trenauny syndrome: Capillary malformation on a leg with underlying LVM, large lateral vein, limb hypertrophy due to bony enlargement.

Koebner phenomenon: Vitiligo induced by trauma.

Kuttner tumor: Chronic sclerosing sialadenitis of the submandibular gland.

Langer's lines: Direction of pull on skin when cut. Least gaping seen when cut along Langer's lines.

Leukoplakia: White keratotic patch on the mucosa that cannot be scraped off. May be associated with intraoral cancer.

Lisch nodules: Hamartomas of the iris.

Long face syndrome: Vertical excess in the facial skeleton. The upper teeth show more than 3.5 mm when the patient is at rest. Narrow alar base and convex nasal dorsum. Recessed chin. Class II malocclusion. Due to increased lower third height.

Lop ear: A malformed auricle in which the characteristic deformity is an acutely down-folded or deficient helix and scapha, usually at the level of the tuberculum auricle. Is often associated with a malformed antihelix, usually at the superior crus.

Maffucci syndrome: Multiple enchondromas and venous malformations.

Mandibulofacial dysostosis: Aka Treacher Collins syndrome.

Marjolin ulcer: SCC at site of chronic scar or inflammation, typically in old burn injuries.

Maxillonasal dysplasia: Aka Binder syndrome.

McGregor patch: Osseocutaneous ligament at the level of the zygoma that acts as one of the retaining ligaments of the face.

Meige syndrome: Dystonic disorder of the facial and oromandibular muscles with blepharospasm, grimacing mouth movements, and protrusion of the tongue usually occuring in older women.

Milroy disease: Lymphatic malformation leading to neonatal lymphoedema.

Missing bone disease: Aka Gorham Stout disease. Intraosseous lymphatic malformations with multiple areas of degeneration.

Möbius (or Moebius) syndrome: A disorder of unknown etiology that involves cranial nerve palsies and limb abnormalities. Typically CN VI and VII but V and VIII can be involved. Sindactyly, brachydactyly, talipes equinovarus, absence of pectoral muscles.

Muir-Torre syndrome: Multiple internal malignancies, cutaneous sebaceous proliferation, keratoacanthomas, basal or squamous cell carcinomas.

Multiple neonatal hemangiomas: Anemia, congestive heart failure, hepatomegaly, multiple cutaneous and hepatic hemangiomas, high mortality rate (~54%).

Nager syndrome: Aka acrofacial dysostosis. Similar to Treacher Collins but more rare. Associated with preaxial hypoplasia or aplasia of upper ± lower extremities. Usually have cleft palate, short stature, and mental retardation. Lid colobomas are rare.

Nevus of Ito: Blue-gray discoloration of the shoulder region, more common among Japanese.

Nevus of Ota: Blue pigmentation of sclera and periorbital skin, more prevalent among Japanese.

Nevus sebaceous of Jadassohn: Aka Nevus sebaceous. Tumor arising from sebaceous glands with a 20% to 30% malignant transformation.

Nikowsky sign: Skin blistering after minor frictional trauma.

No reflow phenomenon: Failure to reperfuse tissue following re-establishment of vascular flow (assuming adequate arterial perfusion and venous outflow).

Oppenheimer effect: Animal study in 1948 that showed implanted metals in experimental animals could induce tumors. Yet to be proven in humans.

Orbital apex syndrome: Neuritis, papilledema, or blindness caused by fracture through the optic canal. Loss of consensual reflex differentiates this from superior orbital fissure syndrome.

Oxycephaly: Sagittal and both coronal suture synostoses. Pointed skull.

Parkes Weber syndrome: Capillary malformation on the arm or leg with underlying limb hypertrophy due to bony enlargement. AV fistula differentiates from Klippel Trenauny.

Parry-Romberg disease: *See* Romberg disease, Hemifacial atrophy.

Patau syndrome: Trisomy 13 leading to changes in the midface, eyes, and forebrain. Microcephaly, wide sagittal sutures and fontanelles, cutis aplasia, microphthalmos or anophthalmos, colobomas, cleft lip and/or palate, low-set ears, polydactyly, heart defects, cryptorchidism. Three-quarters die by one year of life.

Pfeiffer syndrome: Acrocephalosyndactyly II. Coronal synostoses. Tower skull, prominent forehead, flat occiput, orbital hypertelorism with exorbitism, midface hypoplasia with class III malocclusion, high arched palate, and possible submucous cleft. Syndactyly of hands and feet with thumb and great toe wide, short, and deviated medially. Autosomal dominant.

Pierre Robin sequence: Outdated term. See Robin sequence.

Pitanguy's line: Line from 0.5 cm below the tragus to 1.5 cm above the lateral brow that predicts the course of the frontal branch of the facial nerve (deep to temperoparietal fascia).

Plagiocephaly: Distorted skull due to either synostoses or deformation. Can be either anterior or posterior.

Porokeratosis: Autosomal dominant, abnormal keratinization with malignant degeneration.

Port-wine stain: Outdated term for capillary malformation.

Posterior plagiocephaly: Single lambdoid suture synostoses. Twisted skull.

Progeria: Premature aging with growth retardation, baldness, and atherosclerosis. Short life span with rapid disease progression.

Proteus syndrome: Asymmetric overgrowth of bone, soft tissue, nerve and connective tissue and the possible development of vascular malformations.

Pseudoxanthoma elasticum: Increased collagen breakdown and deposits of fat and calcium on elastic fibers, autosomal recessive. Pebbled, lax skin with yellowish papules and no elastic rebound. Also angina, leg aneurysms, hypertension, angioid streaks, and retinal detachment. Safe to operate.

Ramsay Hunt syndrome: Herpes zoster oticus infection leading to facial palsy.

Rendu-Osler-Weber disease: Hereditary hemorrhagic telangectasia. AVM in skin, mucosa, lungs, abdominal viscera. Autosomal dominant.

Reperfusion injury: Event after re-establishment of flow to a flap where free radicals that collected during the ischemic period then contribute to endothelial cell damage, swelling, and increased permeability.

Robin sequence: (Formally known as Pierre Robin sequence) A collection of dysmorphic changes including micro-gnathia (corrects with age), macroglossus with glossoptosis and cleft palate. Associated with multiple chromosomal abnormalities, genetic disorders, and teratogenic influences.

Romberg disease: Hemifacial atrophy. Gradual wasting of one side of the face. Skin, hair, eye, soft tissue, and skeletal atrophy and hypoplasia. Occasional contralateral Jacksonain epilepsy and migraines. Sporadic and questionable etiology. Coup de Sabre lesion is pathonomonic.

ROOF: Retro-orbicularis oculi fat. Preseptal fat pad of the upper lid.

Saethre-Chotzen syndrome: (Previously known as Acrocephalosyndactyly III). Variable synostoses involving unilateral or bilateral coronal suture. Flat forehead and occiput, orbital hypertelorism with exorbitism, blepharoptosis, midfacial hypoplasia with class III malocclusion, beaked nose, prominent helical crura, and high arched palate. Short staure, minor syndactyly, brachydactyly, renal anomalies, mild mental retardation, and cryptorchidism. Autosomal dominant.

Salmon patch: Aka Angel kiss, Stork bite. Macular patch on the posterior neck seen in over 50% of newborns. Flat, pale pink to brown, fade during infancy.

Scaphocephaly: Sagittal suture synostoses. Long, keel-shaped skull.

Schirmer's test: Test of the greater petrosal nerve by measuring tear secretion using filter paper applied to the lower conjunctiva for 5 minutes. Less than 10 mm is abnormal. Schirmer's Test 2 includes the use of local anaesthetic to block reflex tear secretion.

Short face syndrome: Vertical deficiency in the facial skeleton. Edentulous-appearing, short, square face. The upper teeth do not show when the patient is speaking. The corners of the mouth are below the midline. Broad alar base and large nostrils. Due to decreased lower third height and maxillary height.

Shprintzen syndrome: Aka velocardiofacial syndrome. Microdeletion on chromosome 22. Notable features include pharyngeal hypoplasia, severe hypernasality, learning and language impairments, cardiac abnormalities, microcephaly, vertically long face, square nasal root, long philtral column, thin lips, and retruded mandible.

Simmonart's band: Bridge of tissue stretching across the upper lip in a cleft lip.

Sjorgen syndrome: Dry eyes (keratoconjunctivitis sicca), dry mouth (xerostomia), rheumatoid arthritis.

SOOF: Suborbicularis oculi fat. Preseptal fat pad of the lower lid.

Spee, Curve of: Natural curve of teeth in a superior/inferior direction as one moves mesial to distal on the dental arch.

Spitz nevus: Aka juvenile melanomas, epitheloid cell nevi. Firm red-brown nodules, present early in childhood, resemble melanomas on histology.

Stahl ear: Ear characterized by the presence of a third crus that transverses the upper third of the ear.

Stickler syndrome: Commonly associated with connective tissue diseases. Key features include Robin sequence (most common syndrome associated with Robin sequence), cleft palate, and severe myopia, vitreal degeneration, and possible retinal detachment, as well as long bone abnormalities at growth centres, minor spine anomalies, and risk of high-frequency hearing loss.

Stork bite: Aka Salmon patch, Angel's kiss. Macular patch on the posterior neck seen in over 50% of newborns. Flat, pale pink to brown, fade slowly.

Sturge-Weber syndrome: V1 ± V2, V3 capillary malformation with ipsilateral leptomeningeal vascular anomalies. Seizures, glaucoma, retinal changes, low IQ.

Superior orbital fissure syndrome: Exorbtism, ophthalmoplegia, ptosis, midriasis (dilated pupil), V1 anaesthesia.

Synostosis: Abnormal fusion between cranial bones.

Telecanthus: Excess distance between the medial canthi. Must be separated from hypertelorism.

Tinel's sign: Sharp electric-like pain when the leading tip of a regenerating nerve or injured nerve is tapped.

Towering head deformity: Aka turricephaly.

Treacher Collins syndrome: Aka mandibulofacial dysostosis, Franschetti syndrome and confluent Tessier 6, 7, 8 cleft. MENCOP: *M*andible hypoplasia, *E*ar (microtia, cryptotia, middle ear abnormalities), *N*ose (narrow, deviated, hooked), *C*heek (hypoplastic or absent zygoma and macrostomia), *O*rbit (lateral lower lid colobomas, absent medial lower lashes, antimongoloid slant), and *P*alate (high arched/occ. clefted). Autosomal dominant (5q31).

Trigonocephaly: Metopic sutural synostoses. Triangular-shaped skull.

Turban tumors: Large or multiple cylindromas on the scalp.

Turricephaly: Aka Towering head deformity. Bilateral coronal suture synostoses (also causes brachicephaly). High skull.

Van Der Woude syndrome: Cleft lip ± palate with lower lip pits. Occasional absence of 2nd molars. Variable penetrance autosomal dominance with IRF6 mutations.

Velocardiofacial syndrome: Aka Shprintzen syndrome, DiGeorge sequence (10% of patients). Microdeletion on chromosome 22. Most common syndrome associated with cleft palate. Also pharyngeal hypoplasia, severe hypernasality, learning and language impairments, cardiac abnormalities, microcephaly, vertically long face, square nasal root, long philtral column, thin lips, and retruded mandible.

Virchow's law: Growth proceeds (with or without overcompensation) in a direction parallel to the affected (synostotic) suture.

von Recklinghausen disease: Aka neurofibromatosis. Multiple cutaneous neurofibromas, five or more café-au-lait patches greater then 1.5 cm in diameter, axillary freckling, Lisch nodules of the iris.

Wallerian degeneration: Described by Waller. Destruction of distal axons and myelin following transection of a nerve by macrophages and Schwann cells. These collapsed nerves form the bands of Buenger.

Warthin tumor: Adenolymphoma of the parotid gland, typically located in the tail.

Werner syndrome: Adult progeria. Autosomal recessive connective tissue disease with poor wound healing.

Wolfe's law: Bone will form strength along lines of maximal stress.

Wyburn-Mason: Syndromic frontonasal capillary malformation with unilateral AVM of retina and optic nerve.

Xeroderma pigmentosum: Defective DNA repair mechanism leading to multiple epitheliomas with malignant degeneration. Autosomal recessive.

INDEX